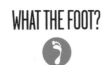
WHAT THE FOOT?

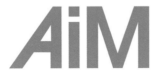

A GAME-CHANGING PHILOSOPHY IN HUMAN MOVEMENT TO ELIMINATE PAIN AND MAXIMISE HUMAN POTENTIAL

BY GARY WARD

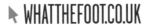

▶ WHATTHEFOOT.CO.UK

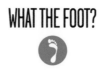

WHAT THE FOOT?

First published 2013 by Soap Box Books

30 Wellington Street, Covent Garden, London WC2E 7BD

www.soapboxbooks.co.uk

ISBN: 978-1-907261-08-4

Printed By Print On Demand Worldwide

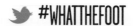
#WHATTHEFOOT

WHAT THE FOOT?

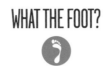

WITH THANKS

To Kai and Isla

For Hamish... may he rest in peace

And my beloved wife, Linzi, without whom none of this would be possible

THANKS TO:

Linzi, Kai, Isla, Mum, Dad and Andrew for their support in my development
and career choices. Isla was only four weeks old when I began writing this book.
Darren Kennedy for putting me on this path.

Julian Mills for first teaching me about feet. Mark Coles for taking me on as a PT all
those years ago. Countless people who have donated their bodies in the name of
my research and development. Mike Weeks who I credit for the name
Anatomy in Motion. Ade Baxter and Oliver Dudley for the AiM video
we made and Stu Metcalf for producing it.

Mik Bjorkenstam for the headshots, we simply swapped a photo session for a new
pair of feet. Not forgetting Dominic Scott who's ability to turn countless black and
white Word docs into the beautiful book you hold in your hands.

A whole bunch of students too many to name, you know who you are, I am
grateful for our interactions, each and every one of you. And finally to Ben
Houghton, without whom this book would never have made it past the first post.
I'm indebted to your support, friendship and commitment to my cause. ☺

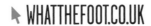

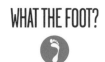

MORE PRAISE FOR GARY WARD

"If you work in the movement industry and want results read this book and learn AIM. Nothing could arm you better than the game changing concepts #whatthefoot brings to life. Light has been shone into a dark place. Thank you Gary Ward for this"
Dr Carlyle Jenkins, Leading Sports Chiropractor, Harley Street

"Gary's philosophy is fresh and unique but ultimately beautiful in its simplicity... it is also devastatingly effective! By applying his methods in my consultations (which are only 10 minutes long!!), I have helped many patients become pain free and already had to cancel one patient's scheduled knee operation!"
Dr Rangan Chatterjee, GP

"This book is a simple MUST read whether you are an athlete, a personal trainer, a physio, chiro or osteo. I feel I have been given a gift from Gary and reading his long awaited book just cements my feelings WTF? Really? Yes it unlocks the potential in everyone."
Lisa Letchford, Olympian, GB Hockey, Beijing 2008

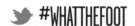

WHAT THE FOOT?

FOREWORD

When I first met Gary Ward on Facebook, I knew this was a person that shared my ideas about how the body worked. In my 40 years of practice, this is a very unusual experience. The first time we met we worked together on a student of mine, each of us not knowing what the other was going to do next. It was like playing jazz, each of us improvising off the other, and the results were outstanding.

Since then, we have studied each other's techniques. We both approach the body as an integrated system whose mysteries can be unlocked if you pay attention to the right details. My approach, NeuroKinetic Therapy™, utilises the brain's reaction to concentric loading. Gary's approach, Anatomy in Motion, utilises the brain's reaction to eccentric loading. These are opposite sides of the same coin.

When I was learning Anatomy in Motion with Gary, I realised what a powerful therapeutic modality it truly is. Experiencing the changes in my movement patterns and in my body when Gary artfully manipulated me with his very creative and innovative technique, made me fully appreciate the incredible system that he has created.

Why does a corrective movement system like AiM add value to other therapies? The beauty of Gary's work is that it addresses movement dysfunction with the client in the position that is the basis for every activity – the gait. I have never seen anyone breakdown the gait in such incredible detail and relate it to the entire body as Gary has. Gary's studies of the mechanics of the foot and ankle are impressive, but his creativity with movements to enhance changes to the entire musculoskeletal system is where his brilliance shines. Furthermore, his ability to teach all of this in a clear and concise fashion makes his classes immediately applicable and fun.

I urge you, the reader, to allow yourself to open your mind to a new paradigm in movement therapy.

David Weinstock
Founder of NeuroKinetic Therapy™ Seminars
Author of NeuroKinetic Therapy™– An Innovative Approach to Manual Muscle Testing

WHAT THE FOOT?

CONTENTS

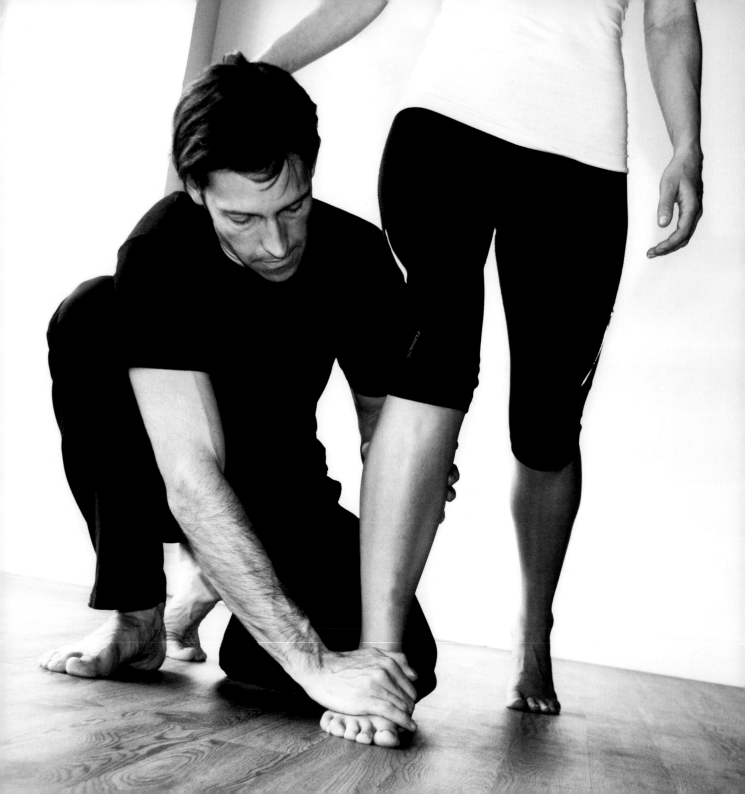

THE END

For me, the end came a long time ago. What I mean by the 'end' is the end of an old way of thinking. The end of personal training, rehab and therapy approaches as they were taught to me (and you). The end of couch-based assessments, massage for rehab and treating the knee when the knee hurts most!

Everything, in fact, that science has strived to prove for the past 300 years must begin to come to an end as we open up a brand new chapter for training, exercise, rehab and corrective processes in the world of human movement. This movement for movement has already begun, but has not yet been fully embraced, and I believe it is the role and responsibility of those who are already transfixed by this way of working to spread the word of the new beginning, a new way of thinking and a new way of giving 'life' back to our ailing clients, patients and the masses around us who merely cope with life as they know it, putting up with pain (need we?), unaware of their bodies (really?), relying on others when things go wrong (sadly)...

The beginning is not much different to the end, just a millimetre or two shift to the right – doesn't seem much now, but in the long run it will be noticeably large. It's time to build on the information that points to this current point in time and build a new path into the future. The outcome in the beginning will be stronger, longer lasting and more powerful than in the end. My book is here to explain to you my reasoning for this and to welcome you into the new beginning. It's an exciting time for anatomy. I hope I can share it with you....

The beginning is not much different to the end, just a millimetre or two shift to the right – doesn't seem much now, but in the long run it will be noticeably large

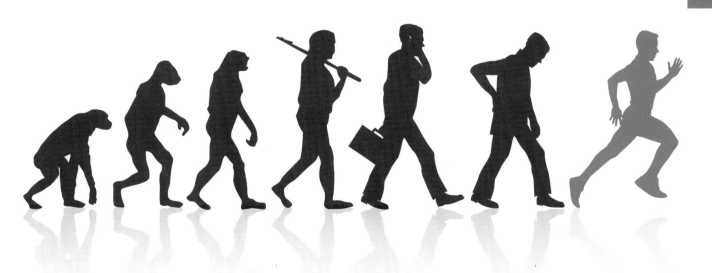

This book is, I hope, the catalyst for your future journeys in the realm of anatomy, exercise, training, therapy and rehabilitation

DEAR READER

I remember going on holiday, aged 21, with a bunch of mates. We arrived at the swimming pool, it looked a bit chilly, one of the lads stripped down to his trunks and was in before you could say calcaneal inversion! The second slipped his shoes and socks off, dipped his toe in the water to weigh up whether he would get in or not and the third kept his clothes on, adamant that there's no way he's getting in today, insisting that the water would be too cold...

But there's always tomorrow!

In writing this book, I am operating from the assumption that you are reading it for one of three reasons:

1. You already have knowledge and experience as a fitness and/or therapy professional, you are fascinated by the human body and have a hunger to know as much as you can. You may be at odds with conventional information or simply just want more. Importantly, you are willing to experiment and learn to become the best you can be and you want to read about movement in a way that will be useful and easy to apply to your professional life.

2. You are working through this book either in preparation for the Anatomy in Motion (AiM) Finding Centre course or you are so close to having made your decision to jump on board and just want as much information as you can while you wait.

3. You are someone who might find that the material presented is a challenge to your existing thought processes and practice, which of course is fine. The wonder and complexity of the human body inevitably produces huge opinion and variation of practice. All I would ask is that you recognise that this is a process based on practical and demonstrable shifts in theory and practice, which can only fully be appreciated through experience. In order for you to take part in this book, I hope it's presented in a way that gently challenges your current thinking and would only ask that you evaluate it through practise and experience as much as debate.

For the purpose of clarity, I would like to address each of the three descriptions above in turn. You may read the one most applicable to you or enjoy reading through all three.

1. Dear budding professional

Like you, my interest in anatomy and the chase to understand it has provided me with a greater hunger than anything else on this planet – apart from, perhaps, the question "Why am I here?" – but at least I have had a glimpse into how we do what we do here, if nothing else.

This book is, I hope, the catalyst for your future journeys in the realm of anatomy, exercise, training, therapy and rehabilitation. The sections of this book are designed to provide you with specific information to help you recognise the value in all that you have learnt so far and the new spaces that it's possible to take this work in your future. Most trainers and therapists leave their base foundational education with a sense of total understanding for the human

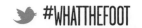

body. You know how to exercise, write programmes, provide therapeutic interventions, treat clients, work with anybody who has a body of their own... Or do you? My specific aim is to create an environment in the pages of this book that will simply challenge the knowledge you have amassed already, wake you up to the comfort zone you have been introduced to and stimulate you to become the best possible practitioner you can be — one who is in high demand and recognised for results and ability to decipher this thing called the human body in the blink of an eye.

I have set the book up to look at some key concepts — things we are led to believe are true — that simply fall flat on their face when we look at the body in motion. The body in motion changes everything. The science we have in our industry to support it is NOT based on the moving body, it's based on dead people and, in a nutshell, it is this that changes everything.

I hope to be able to give you tools to tackle the way you perceive the human body, to facilitate your thought processes when faced with the human body and to fall in love with it all over again. What I have not written this book for is to give you the answers and capability to work with the moving body as I do, as that will take further instruction and time dedicated to the cause. Whilst it's not difficult, it is a challenge to the existing paradigm, so we should tread carefully together into the next phase. I'd love to support you on that journey.

2. Dear future AiM practitioner
As a future AiM practitioner, specialist in the realm of human movement and gait, eliminator of pain and facilitator of peak performance, I salute you for taking the leap required to understand the

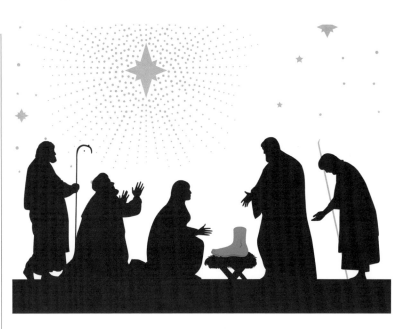

human body from the perspective of a whole new dimension.

You have left behind the comfort zone of what you know, overcome the intrigue of working with the body in motion and stepped into the unknown. Congratulations, the rest is straightforward. In a matter of months you will join an elite group of practitioners making waves in the world of fitness and therapy.

This book now becomes an accompaniment for your journey through the courses, a manual or text book, if you like. Whilst it has been made accessible to everyone, those of you on the Finding Centre journey — or indeed those who have completed the courses and enjoy working with the AiM method already — will read, hear and see between the lines and appreciate the messages on a different level

I hope to be able to give you tools to tackle the way you perceive the human body, to facilitate your thought processes when faced with the human body and to fall in love with it all over again

My intention then, for you, is to soften the areas that lie in between disciplines, suggesting there remains one way within which to work

due to the support and concentration of content throughout the course, which grows deeper at each level until everything in this book appears ultimately simple, straightforward and simply makes sense.

It's highly likely that the book will make most sense when you have completed the course, and it will remain a potential challenge to those who haven't yet taken the leap.

3. Dear potential sceptic?

There's every chance you had this book thrust into your unexpecting arms, rather than seeking voluntarily to engage in its content. Maybe you have heard of myself or Anatomy in Motion, perhaps you've seen or heard of my practitioners at work? It's quite possible that you are sceptical of what you have seen.

That's fine. In fact, it is highly possible that some of the content in the pages that follow might not be on terms with how you currently perceive anatomy, movement and rehab to be. This book is based purely on my experience and the reaction from students and clients alike that suggest what we do and what we talk about works! I, and the people I work with at Anatomy in Motion, consistently aim to challenge the foundations on which it's built to ensure they last and hold true to every aspect of anatomy and physiology.

It could be that if there was to be a reason for you reading this book, it is to take the information on fully before challenging it. I'd invite you to challenge it not with the words that you have heard other people say, nor the words that form the very foundation upon which you base your approach, but on the true and personal experience of how you work and the results

you achieve once you merge the two worlds (yours and mine) together... at that point the challenge will be fair and considered.

My intention then, for you, is to soften the areas that lie in between disciplines, suggesting there remains one way within which to work. Once upon a time, an osteopath declared how very osteopathic my movement–based approach is and in the very same week a chiropractor claimed how very chiropractic my movement–based approach is... I know personally that the pair of them thought each other's work was the work of the devil.

HOW SHOULD I WORK THROUGH THIS BOOK?

From start to finish. In order to structure this book I have assumed you will read the chapters in order. Many of the later chapters refer to ideas, techniques and patterns covered in earlier sections. It will also be advantageous if you take time to pause at the places where it is indicated to do so. Do the tasks and fill out the boxes before moving on.

My intention was to write this book in a style that is as if I am talking to you so that it is as experiential as possible. I hope this is how you will read it.

Lastly, rather than simply read and consciously evaluate this book, I would invite you to experience it as much as possible. At several points within the book you will be asked to imagine, think of an example of or do what is being described. The more you do this, the more you will take from the material.

Please enjoy.

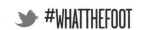

MY STORY

I love feet. In fact, I'm obsessed by them. My anatomical journey began as a ski boot fitter in France. Many a day whiled away on the slopes of Méribel, Les Trois Vallées, with my working hours spent dealing with people's feet and the physical pain they had been experiencing on the slopes that day. Within days of assessing feet, correctly fitting ski boots and building orthotics, two things became clear: 1) we changed the shape of the foot to minimise effort in the boot whilst maximising experience on the ski slope; and 2) the changes down below dramatically impacted on the structures above. It first became clear that adjustments 'down there' made things feel better everywhere, and slowly I realised that a change in the foot seemed to also have the potential to shift the person's pain from one location to another: in the blink of an eye. WTF?

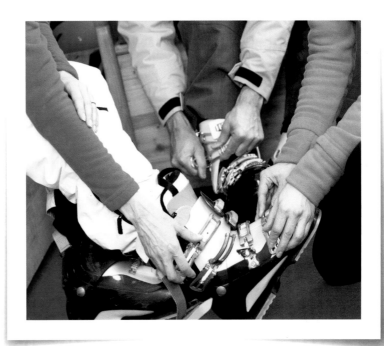

As I qualified firstly as a sports therapist and then a personal trainer (to try and understand the rest of the body better), I was disappointed on two fronts. One, that the knowledge on the foot was weak and, as a result, not discussed; and two, that the integration of foot and body seemed completely unconsidered and overlooked – even though an obvious change in the shape of the foot could change things upstairs, liberate the system and reorganise apparently everything. Like it or not, there is a real and obvious link. Trainers and therapists tend to worry about the ankle and above, whilst podiatrists primarily concern themselves with the knee down, and the integration of it all was missing. Why don't they just team up for God's sake? I started teaching seminars on feet and posture. Everybody loved them. Nobody got it, not even me! But I set my stall out to understand it and the journey from then until now has been amazing.

What the Foot? (#whatthefoot) exemplifies my journey to date. I'd walk into a room full of trainers or therapy professionals professing that the foot can and does influence the whole body and can be a factor in people's pain. Their initial reaction?

WTF?

I've been laughed out of many a room. Most fitness and therapy professionals consider the foot to be at the mercy of the rest of the body, a mere slave

> *Trainers and therapists tend to worry about the ankle and above, whilst podiatrists primarily concern themselves with the knee down, and the integration of it all was missing*

A therapist trained in movement will have an appreciation of full body motion and the interconnection between each and every joint whilst recognising that communication takes place across the whole system simultaneously via the nervous system

joint. I hail it as the 'Emperor', at least in the world of human movement anyway.

Now, I'm not an all or nothing kind of guy. I write this book with full awareness that what happens in the foot can influence the body and whatever is going on in the body will affect the feet. My biggest learning so far in working with the human body is not that this happens both ways, but that it's impossible to separate them (along with many other things). The truth is not that the foot impacts on the body or is affected by the body, but that both the foot and the body are affecting each other simultaneously all the time. Still, there should be no reason to overlook either one, should there?

By the time a client comes into your work environment, the damage is done. A skilled therapist will be able to tell you how to treat the pain and will hopefully have insight into the cause of the problem. A therapist trained in movement will have an appreciation of full body motion and the interconnection between each and every joint whilst recognising that communication takes place across the whole system simultaneously via the nervous system. What this means is you should be able to relate the role of the client's foot to the problem at large.

It just so happens that skeletal malalignments in the body are therefore manifest in the feet, too. Likewise, problems in the feet show up in the body. What if you could treat both the foot and the body simultaneously to get a greater outcome? What if knowing the biomechanics and movement functionality of the foot to the 'n'th degree gave you indescribable insight as to what is happening in the whole body. You'd be interested, wouldn't you?

I told you before, I love feet, I love the body. It appears to work in a way our industry omits to profess, and we dig harder and harder to find some truth about it – and I'm afraid to say that we'll search and dig for ever. I'm obsessed with the workings of anatomy, what causes pain and how your feet carry an imprint – a signature if you like – of what is happening across the whole musculoskeletal system. With that in mind, it pays to get to know the feet better, how they move, and the influence they have up the kinetic chain at each moment in gait will give you new eyes, change your thinking for ever and elevate your ability to work at levels you never previously thought possible.

Studying movement has presented me with five big rules; five rules that so far have lasted the test of time. We challenge them all the time, and they keep coming up trumps. The interesting thing about the feet is that they are the interface between your inside and outside world, the first point of contact with the ground and the first point of communication, which the rest of the body wholly relies on to maximise its performance and minimise (ideally eliminate) pain for good.

You are not designed to be in pain, pain is merely a guidance tool for you to correct course as you roll along this game of life – a kind of biofeedback sat nav system. You have the same body as everybody else. The way you use it and abuse it dictates the viability and vitality you experience from it on a day-to-day basis. When things go wrong, it's natural to look for help and the majority of that help lies in therapies which address exclusively a) the point of the pain or b) the body without considering what the foot is doing during the time the body spends on its feet.

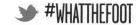

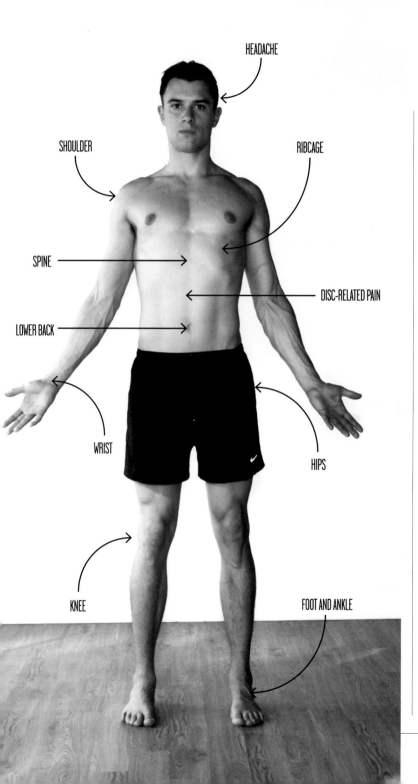

HEADACHE

SHOULDER

RIBCAGE

SPINE

DISC-RELATED PAIN

LOWER BACK

WRIST

HIPS

KNEE

FOOT AND ANKLE

I have direct experience of modifying foot posture without orthotics and directly reducing or eliminating pain in the following places:

- foot and ankle
- knee
- hip
- pelvis
- sacroiliac joint (SIJ)
- lower back – specific and non-specific
- disc-related pain
- spine (upper and cervical)
- ribcage
- shoulder
- wrist
- headache

In each of these cases the pain had been chronic, treated by everybody and deemed as unsolvable for one reason or another. When they came to me, I addressed the feet, addressed the body in motion and had phenomenal impact on the client in less than 60 minutes. Time frames of between one and eight years are classically bandied about to explain how long they have suffered for before they met me. Eight years of knee pain overcome in an hour?

For me, my journey to this point all began with the feet, and today I'm still obsessed with the power they hold over the body.

What, the foot? Really? No way!

WTF?

CHAPTER 1: THE JOURNEY BEGINS

"The journey of a thousand miles begins with one step." Lao Tzu

"You're doing what?" I asked.

"Running seven ultra-marathons in seven days on seven different continents."

I think my next question was "Why?"

When I asked Oliver Dudley how I could help, he told me he had to do it in five weeks' time and he had currently injured his hip to the point of not being able to bear weight on his left leg.

I wasn't surprised to hear that this had happened as a result of him going from zero training to running a straight unprepared 10 miles.

"You're a novice runner as well?" I probed.

"Yes, that's my thing," he suggested nonchalantly. "I was part of the World record-breaking team to row across the Atlantic having never set foot on a boat in my life before!"... and he can't even swim!

My own limiting belief kicked in, though I didn't share it with Oliver, but how the **** was he going to do this event in five weeks' time with little or no preparation. Anyone with two brain cells would most likely prepare a year for something like this. The guy would need a miracle.

So I said "Yes."

At that time it wasn't unusual for me to eliminate somebody's pain in a matter of minutes using the methodology I have developed. That was in March 2009. Since then I have pushed both professional therapists and personal trainers through my training programmes and worked incredibly hard to bring alive the concept that comes so naturally to me: reading and working with the human body... isn't it ironic that my mission is to bring the human body alive? There is, however, a certain truth in that. Never has the human body been so alive, and yet the worlds of fitness and therapy still thrive on evidence based on dead people in an attempt to try and understand how the human body operates.

My mission is simple: to create an awareness of new ways of working with the human body in therapy, performance and coaching circles and bring that alive for fitness and therapy professionals alike – and even the layman, for even he can take control of his own wellbeing, should he choose to.

GROWING PAINS

With a population of nearly eight billion and growing, the world is full of people in pain. Postural distortions, injuries and physical complaints are rife. We have a range of people competing at the top of their game whose daily toil is to stay injury free, and when that policy fails, the question is how quickly can they get back on the field of play?

Thankfully we have a whole industry set up to deal with that; it comprises of therapists such as

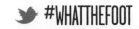

physiotherapists, osteopaths, chiropractors and massage and bodyworkers who work day and night to help you with your pain and problems.

There are also hundreds and thousands of personal trainers, yoga teachers, Pilates instructors, functional trainers, corrective exercise specialists, strength and conditioning coaches and goodness knows what else out there to work on strength, core stability and performance to give the masses access to optimal fitness and wellbeing. If you fit into any of these categories, this book could be for you. I'm going to refer to you all throughout this book as 'fitness and therapy professionals'.

My real question has always been: "With so many fitness and therapy professionals around, all fully trained up, educated to degree standard and seeking continual education, why are so many people still suffering from pain and is there anything else that can be done about it?" The difference, I think, lies in the scientific research and the determination of that research that has, over time, influenced these two industries, establishing the learnings of all fitness and therapy professionals and the methods employed by them to help the masses out of physical strife on a daily basis.

Am I suggesting that current methods don't work? No. Let me be clear, here and now, that that is absolutely not my intention; I will, however, be discussing, based on my experience, some of the potential shortfalls in current methods, as well as bringing to life some of my own theories. Theories, which, in my opinion, act purely as an extension to everything that you, as a fitness and therapy professional, use in your clinical and/or training environment.

My method incorporates full human movement. It's a study of the anatomy in motion and how we (my trained practitioners and I) encourage the body to heal itself through movement. Anatomy in Motion is the name of my business and can be found online at www.anatomyinmotion.co.uk.

I AM HERE TO CHALLENGE YOU!

Some of what I am going to say may challenge your current beliefs and thought processes. Some of what I am going to say may challenge your education and may ultimately have you wanting to throw this book against the wall. Hang in there! My honest belief is that what movement offers you is an extension to everything that is already prevalent in today's therapy world. This means when you add the tool of movement to your existing toolbox the potential for results can only get greater and faster. Unsure? Seek out my own AiM practitioners who are qualified chiropractors and osteopaths who share with me outstanding results having incorporated movement into their own traditional clinic environment.

Also seek out the personal trainers, yoga teachers and Pilates instructors that use this movement-based philosophy in their corrective, rehab and performance programmes. The things these guys are getting their clients to do is unbelievable! What's more, all they are doing is using the medium of movement to create an environment for healing in the bodies of their clients and it's happening in very short time frames for very effective results. What's also incredible is that these practitioners, who themselves are often well qualified, experience huge shifts in their own physical prowess once they add the medium of movement into their own exercise, training and wellbeing programmes.

My honest belief is that what movement offers you is an extension to everything that is already prevalent in today's therapy world. This means when you add the tool of movement to your existing toolbox the potential for results can only get greater and faster

WHAT THE FOOT?

I teach them all to look at the body in a new, exciting and different way. I teach them to read the body, to let the human body give them all the information they need and to give the client's body no option but to heal itself through a deep and profound understanding of the human body.

This new dimension of understanding has been honed into five big rules about human movement that flip conventional anatomy on its head, rip up the anatomy book as we know it and create a whole new handbook and user guide for the human body. Like many new things, it appears complex at first and simple at the end, the more you play and experience the work, the clearer the process becomes.

For now I ask you to park everything you think you know about the human body to one side, out of sight and mind. Keep it somewhere safe as you'll need it later, but for now, in this, the complexity stage, what you think you know now will only hinder any acceptance of what I am going to tell you. It's possible that you'll fight it, deny it, rubbish it, critique it and question it... and yet when you get the chance to put some of it into practice, like many others it's highly likely that you, too, can begin to see the value in this work. Despite everything, it's the practice and experience of it that will ultimately make the difference for you.

WHAT STUDYING MOVEMENT CAN DO FOR YOU

I believe that advancing your skills in any way creates new and exciting opportunities for yourself. When that new skill is as unique and high impact as understanding movement is, there are three natural responses:

A Differentiate yourself
B Be in a position to work with people you can't ordinarily work with and have success
C Grow your business through a unique approach that gets standout, exceptional results

STAND OUT FROM THE CROWD

Training providers are literally pumping personal trainers into your local area on a monthly basis. Pilates and yoga schools are doing the same. Every year, more physios, chiropractors and osteopaths qualify in your area. It gets harder and harder to find work — thankfully there are millions of people looking to get out of pain and get fit, strong and healthy again!

If you are to get noticed in your local area, you must stand out from the crowd. You must differentiate yourself from all the rest. One way of doing that is to learn about human movement for correction and rehabilitation, and three-dimensional training and movement for development and performance.

Right now you are not unique: you choose exercises based on what everybody else is doing. Your packages are unlikely to be bespoke and relevant for each client. I know this because there are apps out there on people's phones offering the same service as you — for free. This is a problem for hundreds of exercise coaches and personal trainers. Apps have become your competitor, too. You have to differentiate yourself from them if you are going to get paid doing what you love. If you only offer standardised training, as most apps do, why would someone pay your hourly rate when Nike offers something amazing for free? Even if you don't think it's amazing, to the consumer it is.

WHAT THE FOOT?

Seek to be different and break the mould of what's expected in your industry. Do this by breaking the mould of your anatomical thinking, understanding and application. Reach beyond what you know and see if there's more to do...

WIDEN YOUR MARKET

You are good at what you do, you are dedicated and proud to be a successful fitness and therapy professional – but can you work with anyone and can you be successful with everyone who comes your way? If you want to help people resolve unsolvable pain, you had better get both the skill set and experience to do so. Following the five big rules gives you direct access to working with some complex and difficult issues whilst seeing incredible results really quickly. I'm not just saying that – there are a whole host of testimonials from clients and happy students that can validate this. When you ask the body to heal itself, anything is possible. The question should simply be: "How can I get your body to help me better understand what is going on?" As you start to get outstanding results, a wide diversity of both goals and problems will begin to seek you out.

FORM AN ORDERLY QUEUE

Both your unique approach in your local area and your unfathomable success with the wide variety of clients that come your way means only one thing: recognition. Recognition brings word of mouth, and success brings people to your door. I get calls on a daily basis asking if I can help people with their pain. The answer is always "Yes!"

When people incorporate human movement in the right way into their business, I have noticed a couple of things: they become a source of intrigue and get more enquiries as to what they do, many of them raise their prices by way of offering a unique product and they become more and more passionate about the work they do based on the clients they attract and the results they see. All this as a result of taking the quantum leap that moves you from being the sheep that follows the herd to being the Pied Piper in your local area.

AS IN THE BODY, AS IN LIFE

One more thing before we venture into the book... You might notice the analogies I make and comparisons I present in relation to anatomy and life. It's a fascinating wonder for me that when I look at and study the human body as a whole inseparable entity, I notice similarities in the life and function of everything from the smallest cell to the big wide universe – recognising that movement itself experiences that natural ebb and flow of polar fluctuations that has huge and significant connotations to the ways of the world and the habits of the human being that are witnessed all around you on a daily basis: in your work, your relationships, your mood, your behaviours and wellbeing, too.

Keep your eyes open for the little hidden messages and see if you, too, can relate the human body to what goes on in your life. I see it everywhere. By understanding the wholeness of the human body I am able to use the principles and the five big rules to help coach somebody through a difficult situation or manage my own family life better. The way of the universe, the way of the world and the way of the human body seem intrinsically connected and inseparable, adding to the richness and fascination that we as beings represent on this planet.

Recognition brings word of mouth, and success brings people to your door. I get calls on a daily basis asking if I can help people with their pain. The answer is always "Yes!"

WHAT THE FOOT?

If you spot this hidden theme, written between the lines, you'll find it easy to get people out of pain and into peak performance on all levels. You'll find it easy to stand out from the crowd. You'll find yourself attracting clients and patients that you previously could not have been successful with, and you'll notice a long line of people queueing at your door to experience first-hand the magical work you are doing with their friends and colleagues.

That is what this book is really about for you: new tools, a greater understanding of the human body, getting superior results with previously unattainable clients and growing a training and therapy business that helps you lead the life you want to lead. Oh, and all of that whilst being true to your passion – discovering the true inner workings of the human body...

Well, it's here, in this book, sewn into the five big rules of motion. I can't wait to share it with you.

A BRIEF HISTORY

Let's assume that we have come to the end of our understanding of traditional anatomy as we know it and through the evolution of practice of that understanding we can naturally start to open new doors for the future. There has always been a ceiling of knowledge we have been approaching and as we approach that ceiling we realise we still don't have all the answers: so there must be something more, mustn't there? New doors like this will always change the way we work and do things.

We got to where we are today with a very simple question: "How does this thing we call the human body work?"

The answer to this question set a framework for the exercises we do today relative to each individual body part and the therapeutic techniques you apply as well.

The problem is that all exercise and therapy theories were created through the study of anatomy, discovering what joints do and recreating that pattern of movement or muscle action into an exercise to stimulate the muscle function, joint range or both.

Firstly, the research into how this body works took place on dead bodies and in an isolated environment and manner – presumably no live volunteers wanted

CASE STUDY

AiM has changed my life, personally and professionally. Personally, AiM has taken my yoga practice and overall mobility to a different level as I now understand why I had any restrictions I did and how to correct this. Even through the late stages of pregnancy I have maintained full mobility and remained pain free. Professionally speaking, I am a completely different yoga teacher. Anatomy training for yoga teachers is often basic or not necessarily up to date. I now teach with confidence, knowing that what I can offer my students will make a difference from the moment they leave the class. As a result, my classes have never been so busy and private work has trebled. I now have this amazing tool to use to help people help themselves, and watching someone go through such a positive, dramatic change after just one simple move is mind-blowing every time. Gary Ward is my biggest inspiration. Tish Dodson www.jivahealth.co.uk

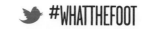

the electrical stimulation caused by the original electromyography (EMG) testing!

This created today's awareness of how muscles work and the impact that muscular contraction has on the joint system.

Secondly, this testing took place in an isolated environment, again, primarily because it's difficult to integrate the body parts of a dead person! The result is that for many years we, too, have been forced to work in an isolated environment: separating body parts to exercise them, and isolating treatments, in particular the areas where people have pain.

There are naturally both major limitations and benefits to this process. It seems to me that whenever we interfere like this, with experimentation, that scientific outcome is split keenly down the middle, separating two truths, like removing the egg from the yolk, calling one good and the other bad, or, in this case, simply omitting a whole other process that is natural, integrated and leads to a huge gap in understanding, on the part of today's benefactor – the trainee or student anatomist and ultimately the client who relies on their knowledge to help them.

The problem is not that the top practitioners aren't aware of this: it's the fact that millions of therapists and trainers are sent out into their industries with little appreciation of that, qualified and let loose on the most phenomenal machine in the world – the human body!

So it was discovered that when a muscle is electrocuted, it is also stimulated to contract or shorten, and when that contraction or shortening takes place, the muscle moves a bone in a specific direction, causing a change in the relevant joint: and the anatomy book was born.

It says that the bicep flexes the elbow and the abdominals flex the spine, which naturally led to the magazines' favourite: bicep curls and sit-ups.

Both of these exercises are prescribed by trainers, adored by the masses and yet can cause negative postural change, which influences pain elsewhere in the body.

The study of anatomy led to a static, isolated and one-dimensional approach to training and therapy and generated the many exercises we are taught to use on our clients and athletes every day. Yet without an understanding of the integrative side of anatomy and movement (the study of live people!) these processes alone will either take too long or lead to problems further down the line – a kind of sweeping it under the carpet approach.

Study of movement = the study of live people!

Should the whole industry be abandoned if every exercise can negatively affect people in that way? No!

We just need to look at the bigger picture, to understand it better and recognise that there are, thankfully, major extensions to the way we work that quickly reinforce conventional treatments and training strategies.

Alone, conventional methods have a place, but combined with movement, to influence the brain,

Without an understanding of the integrative side of anatomy and movement (the study of live people!) these processes alone will either take too long or lead to problems further down the line – a kind of sweeping it under the carpet approach

nervous system and physical structures, the conventional methods will finally begin to add up and make sense.

This is why I created my five big rules of motion.

INTRODUCING CHAOS (COINS HAVE ANOTHER SIDE)

I first had a sense, but now I know, that there is a large part of human anatomical understanding that is missing and, more importantly, that when I, or my students, tap into the part that is missing, there is an undeniable truth that lies beneath it.

I call it the 'other side of the coin' – where most of my opinions appear to oppose and conflict the methods currently being taught. Not a great way of winning friends, I must admit.

However, I should make clear, at this point, that what I am saying and what I am going to pour forth in this book is not in opposition to current methods, but is more of an extension of what already exists. It's simply building onto what we already know to make it more powerful.

You cannot have one side of a coin without the other. Both will always be present, yet one seems to grab the limelight and the other shall be overlooked. Wonderfully, when you put both sides of a coin together, you start to see the bigger picture and greater outcomes become possible. There even arises a third side, upon which both sides of the coin can stand together, solid in the awareness that all outcomes are covered.

Now, I'm not the first person to come onto the scene ranting on about human movement, integration of a wholesome system and the 'treat

the cause, not the pain' approach. Yet movement and integration still fail to be completely present in the world of anatomy.

Frustratingly for me, even current concepts of movement that are rapidly infiltrating the fitness and therapy industry are still heavily focused on the conventional side of the coin, which means, for me, that there remain limitations to understanding human movement and the actual practice of it.

I have a vision where the next step is to see traditional therapies, as well as training and exercise companies, incorporating the full understanding of human movement into their way of working, adapting techniques, getting off the couch – when possible – embracing the true workings of the human body and truly integrating the system as a whole. Bringing both sides of the coin to life, exposing the truth.

The future is confusingly impossible to see. Even on the newer side of the coin, there would appear to be a limit to how we work with the human body, but my feeling is we are a long way off from that, and yet seem so close as well. There are only so many bones, joints, arms and legs to worry about, and understanding the complexity of it all has to be getting simpler – it is getting simpler – but we are not there yet. I do wonder though what would happen to our knowledge and awareness if we brought together all the theories of anatomy, from chiropractic and osteopathic to Pilates and yoga, and wonder often if there lies one simple solution to all of it. Somewhere in the centre...

WHAT THE FOOT?

POLITICS?

The political spectrum of anatomy often sees the chiropractors, physios and osteopaths disagreeing on the treatment style of a patient and in many cases openly in front of the patient as well. This leaves the patient confused and with no idea where to turn next.

Imagine the client being told that money they spent on another therapist was wasted and better spent with you. The poor client does not know whether he is coming or going!

Interestingly, on many occasions in discussion with a chiropractor about my work, I hear them say how very chiropractic my approach is... and in conversation with an osteopath how very osteopathic my method is... So underlying it all is clearly a common theme, yet our perceptions of that theme differ wildly depending on our training, education and experience. Much like religion!

THIS BOOK HAS FOUR INTENTIONS:

- **To raise awareness of what I call the five big rules of human movement – bringing the other side of the coin alive**
- **To give you an insight into what happens when we pay attention to those big rules**
- **For you to recognise the insane importance of understanding foot mechanics and the difference it can make to your work as a practitioner**
- **Answering the question:**
- *   **How do I interpret the body better to get stronger results?**

Underlying all of that, I ask you to start to believe that change is truly possible and perhaps even step into my world for the period of time that you read this book and consider that change really does take only an instant to occur.

It's generally accepted that most pain can be resolved in about six weeks (I'm sure there are variations on that) and we are anchored to that thought. A broken bone takes six weeks – why do we imagine a muscle tear or back pain should take the same?

A six-week process to change isn't really a single change, it's millions of changes taking place on a small scale until you finally perceive that a change has been made in you. Except the type of change I am talking about is the quantum leap from the old to a new physical you...

...from nought to six weeks in just 30 minutes!

Interestingly, on many occasions in discussion with a chiropractor about my work, I hear them say how very chiropractic my approach is... and in conversation with an osteopath how very osteopathic my method is...

WHAT THE FOOT?

It is my experience, on many occasions, that using movement as a tool for rehab has given so many things back to so many people; some claim to have their life back – many of them who had given up on ever being out of pain again. They literally came to me as a last resort and wished they'd found me earlier.

What's the difference between what I do and what they had experienced elsewhere? The difference lies in what I pay attention to and the lack of influence that the conventional model of anatomy has had on me. I'm not blinkered in my approach and never have been.

If it didn't make sense to me, I didn't use it.
I did countless courses that were simply a waste of money, that gave me things to look at, but no solution to offer my client or patient. Movement is still the only thing that makes sense to me. Even the anatomy book we all learn from doesn't make sense to me. If it is accurate, then it's limited in its accuracy and can be expanded on greatly, and yet it remains what we all learn from and use as our 'go to' tool for muscle and joint reference.

It's truly amazing what can happen when you take the raw state of the human body, uninfluenced by text books and old science, and just play with it to see what it can do.

For me, it highlighted significantly different ideas and key concepts that challenge the status quo and impact upon everything from:
- the way we stand to the way we move
- the way we exercise and develop strength and specific conditioning
- the way we can treat clients, receive treatment or even treat ourselves
- whether we choose to be stable or more mobile
- whether you can get out of pain or not

These new ideas and concepts began to come together to form my five big rules of motion, which I'll discuss in detail later.

After the trip, Oliver christened me the 'human horse whisperer' – a horse whisperer being a talented horseman with a remarkable gift for understanding horses, who is hired to nurse horses back to health. Except I do that with humans... and have been referred to as the 'human body whisperer' before now.

UNLOCKING POTENTIAL
Here follows some headings that summarise the approach I both use and teach AiM students to follow to get a result with the human body. Scan it, identify it, solve it... it's how we begin to unlock the hidden potential in every client we see and work with.

● **Scan it**
I watch the body in motion and gait, scanning the body, observing the movement of joints and body, reading for anomalies in muscle balance, stance and posture. I look for what is not happening and compare it to what should be happening.

● **Identify it**
I study the movement to recognise poor or failing

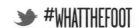

WHAT THE FOOT?

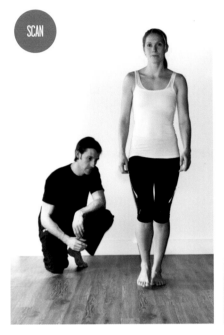

SCAN

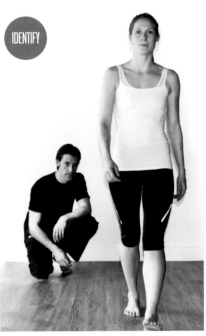

IDENTIFY

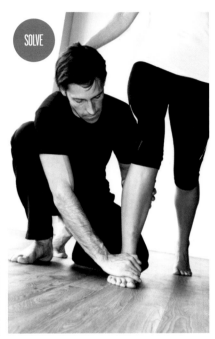

SOLVE

movement patterns so as to seek out and identify the cause of the patient's problem. Poor movement in one part of the skeleton impacts on the movement of the whole skeleton and can be visible from head to toe. I ask myself what movement or imbalance occurring somewhere else in the body could be causing that inhibition.

● Solve it

I use movement patterns, and/or exercises to replace the movement or movements that are not happening in the client's body. These have been mapped to the body over years of watching the body move, and using force and pressure plates to determine how movement occurs from the foot up the kinetic chain. I have developed a way to re-educate the body, to restore lost movement

patterns, which enable the body to function optimally once again. The movement pattern that is faulty (or missing) needs rewiring to the brain so the person can begin to use it again in a pain-free environment.

● Reset

It's like hitting the reset button on an electronic device so the body refreshes itself, starting again, pain free, mobile and raring to go. In fact, this is beyond giving new movement back to the human body. It's about allowing the body to access old movement patterns, the factory setting's default mode. Clearing the decks to start again.

In fact, it is my firm belief that every human body has unlimited potential locked away inside; inhibited possibly by three things:

It's like hitting the reset button on an electronic device so the body refreshes itself, starting again, pain free, mobile and raring to go

---

WHAT THE FOOT?

I. Poor skeletal alignment and posture
II. The internal workings of the body (organ function, hormonal imbalance)
III. Belief or mindset

All of which could have arisen over the years as compensation for previous pain, from postural habit, emotional state, poor attitude to one's health and, of course, present pain or circumstance.

Do we understand pain? Do we respect it? Do we even respect the magical capabilities of the human body itself? I'm not sure en masse that we do.

Let's look at it like this:
If your body is not as good as it can be then it's likely you will have problems at some time in your life.
That much, I think, we all do understand. So if we flip that in reverse (I'll do a lot of that through the book you'll notice) then it becomes:

As soon as your body is as good as it can be, you overcome these problems and create awesome opportunity for yourself.
What I am suggesting is that as overall inhibitions are removed from your body, the overall potential of your body increases, too.

Let's use back pain as our analogy here, since it is the number one search term on Google for the health and fitness industry – notice that people do also seek fitness trainers to help with back pain.

Is this because back care is inadequate? No, it just means that people are always looking for more answers and consistently seeking alternative opinions about their predicament. Human beings thrive on choice. The predicament arises out of the

problem, which is, quite simply, that pain, under the current way of addressing it, is little more than manageable. We have the skill set to help people relieve pain, but do we have the skill set to eradicate that pain for ever? It's an interesting thought. I'd like to create that as a possibility for mankind.

What I am used to witnessing is that people who suffer from back pain can come right out of their pain **immediately** once the overall inhibition has been resolved.

Immediately? How can back pain be the number one search term on Google and therefore the biggest physical problem on the planet if an immediate turnaround is possible?

Quite simply, because it is. On the other side of the coin there is a solution to every problem, and I would like to reveal some of the methods I use throughout this book to give you a basic understanding of how that is possible. So that next time you have back pain and seek treatment, you might think twice about just getting a 'back rub' or a 'back crack' when in reality that could simply be a way of masking the situation in the short term. Next time you consider referring a client for treatment, consider that using movement correctly, as introduced in this book, you could offer a solution where others offer a mask. People need real answers to their pain and real solutions to overcoming performance inhibitions.

Have you ever noticed how every six weeks to three months patients are back at the local therapist with yet another bout of back pain? This is because the environment in which the pain arose has not been challenged or changed. By this I mean the skeletal alignment, the gait patterns, the thought processes

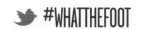

around the pain and the system as a whole remains as it was the last time the pain was present.

It is because change hasn't really happened or even been addressed.

What if it really is as simple as finding the cause, locating the 'thing' that triggers it every day and restoring effective movement patterns to reduce and eliminate the triggers in order to unlock some of that hidden potential I am talking about?

In your body lies an unexplored point of maximum efficiency and optimality beyond which fantastic opportunity lies.

This opportunity can be described as:
- Physiological: a state of enhanced wellbeing, whether it's being pain free and playing with your children or experiencing life at a higher level than you ever thought possible.
- Physical: a perfectly vital body can achieve anything, sporting greatness or just greatness in your own mind. What's your wildest dream?
- Emotional: postural change has an instant carry over to the way you feel and many people remark on the impact that being out of pain has on their life, their family and relationships around them.

This point of maximum efficiency becomes accessible when we challenge the boundaries of what the body can do. There's a weird science, if you like, that makes it simple and easy to compare what goes on in the body to the very nature of how we manage ourselves in life as well.

CHALLENGE
Have you ever noticed how life gets better when you challenge yourself? When you go beyond your own perceived boundaries and self-imposed limitations there is an awareness of change, instant change and a knowing that there is no going back.

Imagine you have pain somewhere in the body. Now imagine that a separate body part simply doesn't work as it should and imagine that challenging and mobilising that part in a specific way means that change at the point of pain becomes a real possibility, with relief instantly brought to your discomfort.

Once you experience that, and feel it in your body, you have a knowing that there is a way out of your current predicament. And there is...

What would you do then? What if all of a sudden there was no pain? What dreams could you fulfil? What goals could you achieve? How different and much more positive would your life be? If you are thinking that you don't know or have run out of dreams or can't even imagine being out of pain, then you have to now seek movement as a tool because it is the one thing that nearly all practitioners and even trainers fail to use in the treatment of your pain. If you have tried everything, but not tried movement, and movement is as effective as I say it is – then what have you got to lose?

Now, as a therapist, consider that your clients feel like that, too... and the best most can offer them is pain management when pain resolution is a real possibility simply by adding new tools – the tool of movement – to your fantastic repertoire of skills. Would you be proud of your work if you knew that resolution was actually possible and yet management is what you are selling?

> *What if it really is as simple as finding the cause, locating the 'thing' that triggers it every day and restoring effective movement patterns to reduce and eliminate the triggers in order to unlock some of that hidden potential I am talking about?*

WHAT THE FOOT?

Your body is being truly functional in its dysfunction!

MOBILITY

One of my biggest fears has always been to lose mobility and as I explore more and more the simplicity of optimising human movement potential, I question how it can be that we are, in the main, happy to have our bodies operate with sub-standard performance.

Why do we accept our pain as the norm and forget to question things until the only possible solution is to be cut open and have parts removed or added to our already perfect body?

You have all the parts you need, ladies and gentlemen!

Yes, your body is perfect, even if you think it isn't. As I mentioned already, not many people truly respect the potential of the human body, including practitioners I speak to and teach. We are forever using the word 'dysfunctional' to describe a failing body. Yet your body is being truly functional in its dysfunction! We'll clear some definitions around this later.

Consistently, when this situation of accepting our pain as normal arises, nobody ever asks: "Have you tried using movement as a tool?" swiftly followed by: "Give your body a chance to heal itself. You didn't know that your own body knows best, did you?"

People are generally left asking the question: "What's happening to me?" and that is the question that I consider on a daily basis: "What is happening in your body that is causing your pain?"

My body knows best? Yup. Despite what your conscious mind is thinking right now, and I accept

that this might be difficult for some of you, but bear with me for now, OK?

Your body has an innate awareness that intuitively knows what it means to work efficiently and effortlessly. It knows how to be pain free if only you would **stop using it in the same way** day in day out and with every step you take. Seriously, changing your body to a more vital state could be the biggest habitual trait you will ever try to break. Harder than smoking. Worse than picking your nails. More debilitating than your need for a biscuit... Unless you get the right type of practitioner in place — one who asks the question "what is happening in your body that is causing your pain?" and understands how to start the process of self-healing or auto-correction, unlock the secrets and crack the code of the human body. Did I mention using movement?

That's what Oliver did. He found me. He paid for me to experience this magical round the world trip because, in Oliver's words, "he couldn't do it without me".

The truth, as he was finding out, is that, sadly, he could not have done it with conventional therapy backing his corner.

MY STORY

I'd like to wind back a bit further to my own story. A trainee teacher with a degree in Modern European Studies at Loughborough University, I spent my years at university gazing out of a window or with my head stuck in my mate's sports science manuals trying to work out how to do better in the gym, build great muscles and wow the ladies. I'd lost the desire to teach foreign languages to schoolchildren who barely even left their home town and thought France

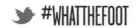

WHAT THE FOOT?

was a fictional land somewhere in the region of Timbuktu. I quit and headed to the Alps to pursue my love of skiing. During the six winters I spent in the French Alps, I was lucky enough to be taught to fit ski boots for a living and even more lucky to be introduced to the foot, how it works, how to fit it in a boot, how to build an orthotic for it, how to make it comfortable and pain free so as to maximise the ski experience of the person at the other end of the body.

I was hooked, instantly. I fell in love with feet and was instantly fascinated with the bodies of the people I worked with. Knee pain, hip pain, back pain: everyone who came in the door had something wrong with them! I remember thinking: "WHAT A BUSINESS!"

Knee pain? What if I adjust the foot in this way? Pain gone? Brilliant; go and enjoy yourself. This happened time and time again. WTF? I also noticed that I could shift pain around from one body part to another, leading me and the other ski boot fitters to question "what is and where is pain really?" We simply deduced it must be in their heads and carried on with our off-snow labour of love: ski boot fitting and ski sales.

Eventually it became too much, I had to learn more and the easiest and simplest way was to become a personal trainer and sports massage therapist. Upon my return to England to work full time in this business I was instantly disappointed with the standard of anatomical understanding in the body – in particular around feet and the phenomenal connection they have with the rest of the body. In fact, I figured people actually believe that the foot and the body are disconnected, like some metal bar sits between the two, separating them and

banning any thought processes that could link the two! There was only one thing to do: start teaching foot and posture workshops. So I did... Today I am lucky enough to teach all manner of fitness and therapy professionals and am constantly honoured by their delight in my approach and humbled by the results they themselves obtain with their clients. I'm passionately driven by the daily feedback I get from my practitioners of the awesome results they get with their clients where other therapists have failed.

This book comes at you with no doctorate, no degree, no background that marries up other than pure experience and practice of working with the human body using the foot as a pure access point to understanding it and determining its functionality. It's been an interesting journey, one that has been fraught with mistakes, errors, struggles and frustrations... but I got there in the end. Following my passion – firstly for skiing, and secondly for the human body – opened doors I hadn't even envisaged when I was sat there feet up staring out the window of Rutherford Hall, Loughborough University, whiling away time in a degree I would barely ever use.

Knee pain? What if I adjust the foot in this way? Pain gone? Brilliant; go and enjoy yourself. This happened time and time again. WTF?

CHAPTER 2: RANT, RANT, RANT!

"Get your facts first, then you can distort them as you please." **Mark Twain (1835–1910)**

Before moving onto the five big rules I first would like to share some of my struggles and frustrations that may also ring a bell with you and your own frustrations. These are things that are prevalent in the businesses and ideologies of fitness and therapy professionals. It's a good time to remind yourself to park what you know and entertain the idea that what I am saying could have some validity and a significant role to play in the way you work with the human body in the future.

When I teach my courses, I get the students to stumble upon these concepts by themselves: that way they can't really disagree with them as they have simply discovered it for themselves. I don't want you just to accept what I am saying – I want you to go out and experience it, play with it yourself and see what happens. Most of all, challenge it and observe the outcomes. The reason I call them the five big rules is because rules are made to be broken and all progress relies on the breakdown and rebuilding of things. I consistently challenge the rules and as yet they remain intact, so I urge you to do the same – don't accept them, run them into the ground and see if they work all the time to serve the people of this world better.

If you finally decide to accept the five big rules, you will most likely notice that in movement, many of the strategies you employ readily in your day–to–day work actually don't carry any functionality or

specificity (two massive buzzwords) across to your client. Wouldn't that be frustrating?

I have 10 basic rants that seem to completely go against the grain of all that we are taught about the human body... and yet when I go against the grain in practice I see amazing transformative results... and so do my students.

RANT #1: STATIC STRETCHING

My core statement here is simple: "Static stretching does NOT work!"

It's quite simple actually. I have not employed static stretching with a client for at least six years now. This MUST mean two things: 1) stretching is not necessary to get results; and 2) there must be a better way than stretching to get the type of results I am used to seeing. The problem, for me, lies in the term 'static'. I don't have a problem with stretching as long as we stretch a muscle in accordance with its true functionality.

Muscle function basics
In motion, all muscles work like so:
OFF – ON – OFF – ON – OFF – ON – OFF –ON
Never static – ever!

To hold a stretch deprives the muscle of the ON part of that relationship. A muscle lengthens to its end range (stretches), stabilises and contracts back to where it started again.

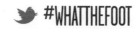

WHAT THE FOOT?

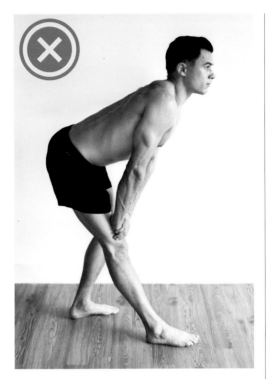

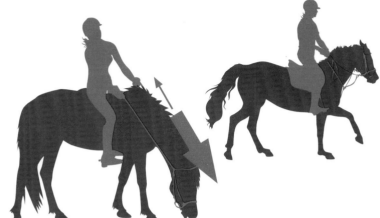

The sensation you feel at the end of a stretch and the reason you can't stretch any further is because the muscle is actively contracting against you. It is defending itself from going too far by decelerating the journey towards end range.

At end range, the muscle has a need to contract back to its restful position, otherwise it will quickly become fatigued in its futile effort to do so.

In movement, muscles stretch to allow the skeleton to move. I call it the 'horse's head' analogy. Imagine you are on a horse, holding the reins, and the horse drops its head to the ground. You are the nervous system that senses that motion and initiates a contraction on the reins to control the movement of the horse's head. If the horse was much stronger than you and placed its head on the floor to eat, and you maintained the effort of trying to get the head back up, you would tire yourself out. This is the case in a static stretch.

When it came to riding the horse minutes later, the horse would be ready to go and you would be knackered! This is how muscles feel in poor posture – knackered.

In dynamic movement, muscles BOTH lengthen and shorten, lengthen and shorten, off – on, off – on. By encouraging this pattern, the body naturally allows the short muscles to lengthen and the overstretched muscles to shorten as the body finds a natural state of balance.

Stretching simply addresses the inhibitions in muscle tone without addressing the state and balance of the body as a whole. In my second big rule of human movement, you will see why expecting a stretch to influence posture is a hopeful long shot at best.

If the horse was much stronger than you and placed its head on the floor to eat, and you maintained the effort of trying to get the head back up, you would tire yourself out. This is the case in a static stretch

RANT #2: SEPARATING ECCENTRIC AND CONCENTRIC ACTIONS

Normally, everybody understands these terms:

Eccentric movement = muscle lengthening under load
Concentric movement = muscle shortening under load

As a result of electrocuting bodies in the name of research, we have been so focused on the concentric shortening action of muscle. And in some cases we focus on the eccentric lengthening of a muscle, but rarely do we consider the fact that concentric and eccentric actions come as a pair – an inseparable pair whose opposing functions actually work together.

By working the two together and not in isolation, the brain, nervous system and the muscles begin to re-understand what the true role is of muscles in movement and daily life. Take a good look and you'll notice that no animal on the planet contracts its muscle before it lengthens. Watch carefully. Understand the rules. Human beings are no different.

I want you to take this moment to notice that if concentric and eccentric actions work together to enhance the role of muscle, why would we ever, in reality, consider using only one part of this story?

What about isometric?
I always get asked this question. Isometric training could be my third rant, but I don't want to sound too much of a whinger. In actual fact, I love isometric

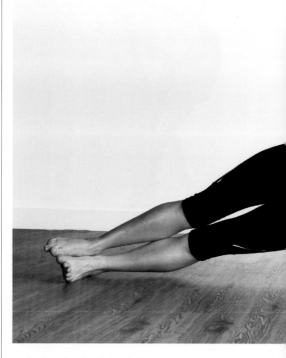

work, timed perfectly in relation to the eccentric and concentric actions of muscle.

Put simply, isometric actions just need to happen at the right time. Standing there holding a pair of dumb-bells out to the side in the name of isometric training, or holding a plank for a minute or more, is isometric work for sure, but the timing of the isometric contraction is so far out from where it would naturally occur that there is absolutely zero

WHAT THE FOOT?

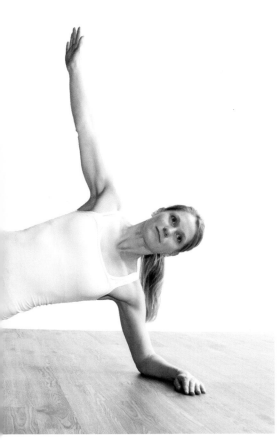

carry over to your movement, your posture or your health.

If you are doing the plank to break a record, then fine, but if you are doing a plank with the goal of strengthening your core, then there are more effective ways of doing so. Quicker, more beneficial and more fun ways of doing so. In fact, I'd stick all movement training into that category — quicker, more beneficial and more fun.

Isometric means that the muscle is neither lengthening nor shortening under load. Have you worked it out yet? The isometric state of a muscle naturally occurs IN BETWEEN the eccentric and concentric action at the point where the muscle reaches its maximum range. This is where you should plan the isometric movement into your training programmes.

How long does it last for?
Less than 0.01 of a second, so is there any point holding it for well over a minute? Not in my book. Add to this, just briefly, that when stretching a muscle statically, you are also holding that position for way too long since access to isometric muscle action is so minimal in real time.

My final point on stretching: stretching a muscle in isolation also breaks down when we look at movement and how, in fact, large groups of muscle lengthen simultaneously, never individually and certainly not in isolation. There is a reason for this and we must NOW begin to understand why.

To begin with, entertain the idea that your brain has no clue what you are attempting to do to it when you utilise a static stretch, train isometrically or focus on concentric actions without coupling up the eccentric part of the movement as well.

If you stretch the hamstring on the floor and then ask me to walk away after our stretch session, the information received by the brain in the stretch from the hamstring, and the information received by the brain when the hamstring is walking, is completely different. One is being held statically for a period of time and the other is experiencing eccentric, isometric and concentric actions coupled with a

If you are doing the plank to break a record, then fine, but if you are doing a plank with the goal of strengthening your core, then there are more effective ways of doing so

WHAT THE FOOT?

> *"Changing something on an upper level changes things on the lower levels; changing something on a lower level could but would not necessarily, affect the upper levels."*
>
> (Dilts, Epstein, Dilts, 1991, p26)

complex array of interconnected muscle and joint actions. So what's your goal?

Stretching has become a way of managing injury and tightness in the body. However, we aren't asking the question as to why the tightness or injury is there in the first place, are we? If we are, and the answer we are coming up with is because the hamstring is tight, then fine, but in this case we need to learn to ask better questions to get better answers and better outcomes, because in truth the relationship between the eccentric and concentric actions operates on a much higher logical level than an isolated aspect of that.

Higher logical levels

www.neurosemantics.com/meta-states/greater-flexibility-using-the-other-logical-levels

"In our brain structure, language and perceptual systems there are natural hierarchies or levels of experiences. The effect of each level is to organise and control the information on the level below it. Changing something on an upper level changes things on the lower levels; changing something on a lower level could, but would not necessarily, affect the upper levels." (Dilts, Epstein, Dilts, 1991, p26)

Integration of a whole system filters down to the individual parts of that system. I work on the whole body and naturally impact upon and benefit the parts of that body, whereas, traditionally, we are taught to work on the parts of the body in the vain hope that we will benefit the whole.

Clients often inform me that they have had their ankle, hip and cervical spine treated. But with a little

questioning, I discover that they were treated in isolation and on a couch.

Using movement as a tool would treat the same body parts in a closed chain environment to benefit all of the joints together and in motion.

The logical levels in the human body might look like this ➜

The higher up the levels you target your practice, the greater impact you will have on the system as a whole. If your work focuses on muscles and joints exclusively through training, massage or joint manipulation, what level of long-term impact can you really have?

Is there reason to isolate anything? Sure there is, but the sooner we move to an integrated place and move up the logical levels, the greater and longer term the outcome will be.

BRAIN

NERVOUS SYSTEM

WHOLE BODY

SKELETON

FASCIAL SYSTEM

JOINTS

MUSCLES

Next time you exercise your mid-section, do you want to focus exclusively on the concentric phase for the abdominals (low logical level) or incorporate concentric, isometric and eccentric actions (high logical level) into your workout? Have a think about it... In the same vein, working on a single dimension of a muscle is a low level compared to the full three-dimensionality of that muscle, which is naturally a higher logical level.

RANT #3: CORE STABILISATION

I was at a talk recently when a physio of a leading football club claimed that the concept of core stabilisation has purely been a marketing fad. A concept invented by some strength and conditioning coaches to make the spine and your back safer.

In actual fact, to be able to stabilise the core is definitely useful in a static, heavy-lifting environment and does carry some benefit for clients and patients with back pain. My rant is simply that to teach the core to stabilise is exactly the opposite from what it should be doing in a normal, healthy human being. So perhaps there is another, better way?

Later, when I introduce the second big rule of motion, I'll explain how we can prove — and I start every course like this — how the body cannot be still, EVER. It is constantly on the move, constantly in motion, and, ironically, when I ask people to stabilise and be as still as possible, they actually begin to move more! How does being stable mean more movement? Being stable actually increases the EFFORT in the physical system, along with joint motion limitations and conscious activations. To be mobile or have mobility available in the system reduces that effort and makes life easier.

Effortless...

Naturally, underneath 450kg of squat, I don't want to be too mobile: so herein lies the value of having a stable core. But a stable core without an awareness of how to be mobile ultimately means that we risk injury and pain and problems further down the line. It may even be that we are teaching ourselves to be stable in an unbalanced position, which is not going to help matters either.

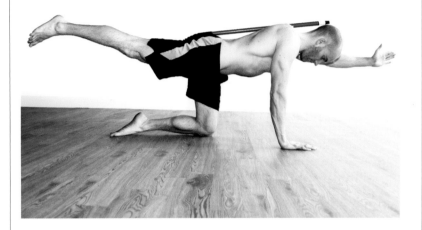

'The body cannot be still, EVER'

In my experience, very few people are naturally well balanced and to spend time stabilising people in their unbalanced posture and stance is not a healthy thing to do since imbalance would appear to be a precursor to our problems and the very thing that movement as a therapy seeks to change.

Imbalance alone is not a cause of injury and pain — there are other motion-orientated components that make injury and pain a certainty.

On a higher logical level, both stability and mobility would be present in each joint to maximise human potential and minimise pain.

So for now, think less core stability and more core mobility... because you can't be stable anyway!

WHAT THE FOOT?

RANT #4: ONE-DIMENSIONAL TRAINING

Another hand-me-down from the research teams of yesteryear is one-dimensional training. This is training or exercise where you look into the mirror and lift some weight without moving your torso, being still and stable, and those who are 'in the know' are hanging on to 'neutral spine' for dear life, and for those that aren't, anything goes as long as the weight and the numbers on those weights goes up!

This is the worst type of exercise you can do for a human body that is CRAVING movement in a three-dimensional space. These exercises would target one dimension at a time, such as a flexion/extension exercise only or a rotational exercise only, occasionally haphazarding, by chance, over a bi-dimensional movement. Your skeleton is free to move in all three dimensions and it's free to do this for a reason, to be able to withstand the forces exerted on it from the outside world. Why limit that by accessing one out of three?

When we teach the human body to utilise each and every joint in the planes of movement available to it, it will naturally improve in all areas of strength, balance, posture, alignment, speed and technique as well as contributing to pain reduction and reducing the risk of future injury, too. One-dimensional exercise might give you big muscles, but it reduces flow and movement in the body, downgrading posture. If you value muscle size over posture and mobility, stick with one-dimensional training. If you want muscle, posture and mobility, why not learn to combine the two?

A quote from T Harv Eker, author of *The Millionaire Mindset*, says: "Rich people think 'both'. Poor people think 'either/or'.", suggesting the sooner you start

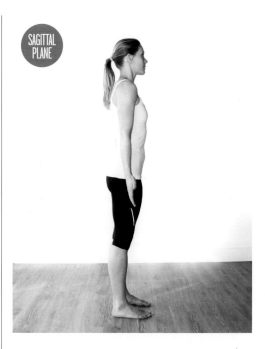

SAGITTAL PLANE

choosing both instead of being torn between two, the richer you will become.

In the human body always choose both or more... and never one as you are limiting any dormant possibility within you and your clients. Seek stability and mobility, seek strength and balance, seek pain-free and high performance!

You won't regret it...

3D

On that note, I should introduce the three anatomical planes of motion for any of you who may be unsure of their specific meaning, as the terms will freely be used throughout the whole book. Each plane of motion can be considered a single dimension of the

WHAT THE FOOT?

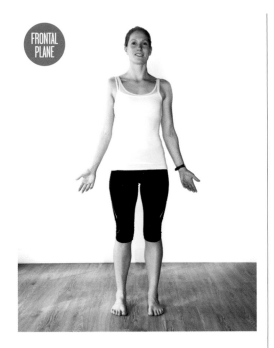

FRONTAL PLANE

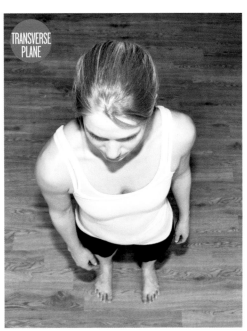

TRANSVERSE PLANE

← GET TO KNOW YOUR ANATOMICAL PLANES AS THESE TERMS WILL BE USED THROUGHOUT THE BOOK:

Sagittal plane
Side on
Frontal plane
Front on
Transverse plane
Top down

three dimensions in which human beings operate. The 1D motion that I am referring to in rant #4 is the sagittal plane motion – primarily flexion and extension. The two oft-forgotten planes in the 1D world are the frontal plane – primarily adduction and abduction – and the transverse plane – primarily rotational motions.

Today, the knowledge of the planes is commonplace and many people simply need reminding of them. To get to know them deeply and recognise that each joint motion has access to one or more of these planes in simultaneous moments is the key to getting to grips with motion-based anatomy. The foot accesses full 3D and sends waves of influence up the whole body, causing three-dimensional chaos in the whole system.

For those willing to hear it at this point, and those who think the body moves in a multi-dimensional way, I think it's important to note that any motion can be broken down into aspects of the three planes of motion. A scapula, for instance, will move partially into each plane and possibly be dominant in one. So it's rarely ever purely in one plane or another, but borrows increments of movements from each and thus can be described positionally in space. A 1D approach for the scapula will never satisfy it of its full potential.

WHAT THE FOOT?

RANT #5: RECIPROCAL INHIBITION

Following on from this is the term 'reciprocal inhibition'. Reciprocal inhibition describes muscles on one side of a joint relaxing to accommodate contraction on the other side of that joint.

It's certainly an interesting one and we have it to thank for the isolated workout programme design. You know the one: chest and back; biceps and triceps; forearms and calves...

You don't have to let go of this one too much as it can be very useful if you are learning to work with the body, but if you want to take your knowledge into the next dimension, then you should recognise that in very few cases during human movement is reciprocal inhibition, as we know it, present at all. In fact, it happens in a far less obvious guise.

Only in single planes can we see evidence of it. In a three-dimensional model it's surprising how many so-called 'opposing muscles' actually play the same role as each other in controlling a movement. I'm sure you can think of a few agonist/antagonist relationships in the foot, hip and torso, and you will be as surprised as I was to discover that they don't really exist when you study the body in movement.

Think erector spinae and rectus abdominus: one flexes and one extends, naturally opposing each other, and yet both of these muscles have identical roles in managing the movement of the spine in the frontal and rotational transverse planes — as do the obliques, quadratus lumborum and latissimus dorsi, albeit with different degrees of force and pull. Have you ever wondered what happens to these muscles when the spine is flexed, rotated and laterally flexed?

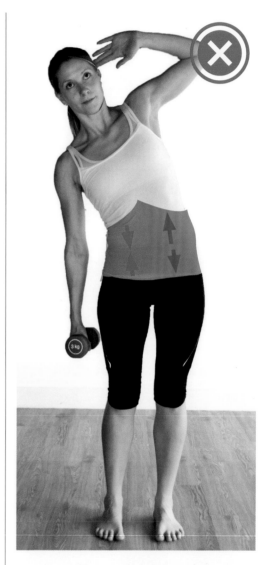

↑ RECIPROCAL INHIBITION OF SIDE MUSCLES IN A LATERAL FLEXION EXERCISE, INCLUDING QL, ABDOMINALS, ERECTOR SPINAE AND LATS. GREEN FOR LENGTHENING AND RED FOR SHORTENING

Doesn't this eliminate the idea that when one is active, the other is inactive? It's completely untrue. There is evidence of this all over the body, especially in the spine and the foot — two key areas on either side of the coin for managing potential in the body.

In addition to this, I feel it a suitable time to let you in on the fact that a single muscle can play different roles in different dimensions at the same time. This means it can be lengthening in one plane and shortening in another plane at the same time. Crazy? Try and put your psoas muscle into a stretch in the sagittal and transverse planes and shorten it in the frontal plane. This happens in one particular phase of gait and actually allows another major muscle to fully stretch in all three planes. Can you work out which one?

So you see, all muscles do what they have to do to allow efficiency and effectiveness in other areas of the body.

Muscles also react to the skeleton, as you'll see in big rule #2, so wherever you place your skeleton will dictate whether a muscle is long in one, two or all three dimensions, whilst being short in the remaining dimensions (two, one or none).

Crazy? Welcome to the eye-opening world of human movement.

Still with me? Write down what you have learned so far. Any questions, tweet me on #whatthefoot.

RANT #6: LOCALISED TREATMENT

Localised treatment is like shining a laser onto the area that is painful as opposed to radiating light from a light bulb over the whole body. Localised treatments focus on a sore knee rather than target the cause of that knee pain. This should be where you, as a practitioner, ultimately want to take your practice, understanding the body as a complete system, otherwise you could get swallowed up in an industry that is rapidly cottoning on to the fact that movement and a whole-body approach gives access to rapid and long-lasting results.

Is it possible you are looking in the wrong places?

A localised approach is rarely the way forward: problems in the back can be caused by poor mobility of one foot, knee problems may be a lack of communication between the hip and the ankle, and a sore neck could be the culmination of poor posture. A stretch in the neck or a simple massage cannot get to the root of this problem — unless the cause actually resides in the neck, of course. Even then, I wonder what the impact would be on the system as a whole.

When we teach the human body to utilise each and every joint in the planes of movement it has available to it, and in perfect synchronicity with the rest of the joints in the system, we increase the functionality of the system as a whole.

Perfect synchronicity here means that the joints have the potential to work together. When joint a does x, joint b does y and joint c does z.

> *When we teach the human body to utilise each and every joint in the planes of movement it has available to it, and in perfect synchronicity with the rest of the joints in the system, we increase the functionality of the system as a whole*

WHAT THE FOOT?

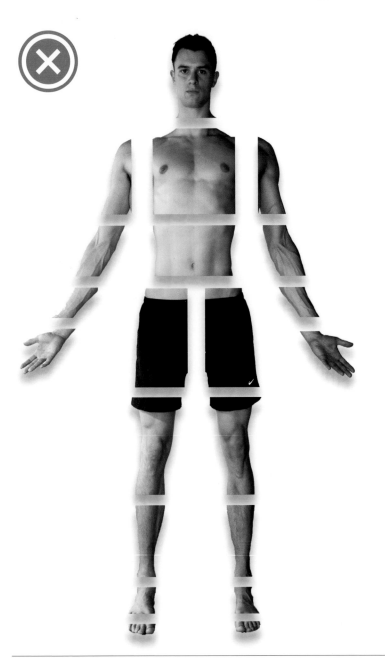

In this sense the whole is far greater than the sum of the parts. We cannot move any part of the human body without affecting all of it at once. This concept is increased and much more visible when we are on our feet. No part of the human body is static when it is in motion – it's all moving at once in one large, free movement.

Isolated treatments aim to increase the functionality of one area at a time in the vain hope that it will impact on the whole system.

When I work with the whole body, I have the intention of re-educating the system to work systematically, by enhancing the communication between all joints and enabling all muscles to operate in accordance with the joint system in a dynamic environment. What I notice is that this process actually does impact on the whole system.

It simply teaches the body to rebalance, eliminating pain and inhibition instantly.

That's what I do and teach, and whilst that might sound a bit much right now, I hope it will become clearer as you go through the book. Time to put your laser away and get the light bulb out?

←THE HUMAN BODY IS WHOLE AND COMPLETE AND YET WE TREAT IT LIKE IT IS A BUNCH OF PARTS, SEPARATE, DISCONNECTED AND ISOLATED

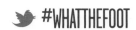 #WHATTHEFOOT

RANT #7: FORCED OR CONSCIOUS ACTIVATION

I actually think we are guilty of forcing change on our clients and patients. We do this by requesting conscious activity in the exercises we prescribe. For instance, asking someone to sit up straight or stand taller is a short-term fix. The person can only initiate it when she thinks about it and naturally forgets about it when she has other things to do. You'll know this, as a fitness and therapy professional who always harps on about posture – I can guarantee that the only time all week that your client stands up tall is when he/she sees you, and you'll actually see him/her move from slumped to upright as soon as his/her eyes catch sight of you.

The information available on brain processing and speeds is varied. However, in general, it is understood that the brain can consciously only process tiny amounts of information at one time.

In a subconscious environment, the brain can process millions of bits of data at one time (everything from remembering a list of to dos, to dealing with the wobbly pavement, to making sure little Jonny doesn't run into the road, to sensing the air temperature, initiating a shiver and making sure you don't bite your tongue in the process). What was that about posture again?

This conscious approach to physical change, then, means that we cannot maintain it full time. How do we think about standing tall, drawing the transverse-abdominis (TVA) in, putting one foot in front of another whilst squeezing my butt at the right time when I do – just like my therapist showed me; all

whilst fumbling in a bag for the car keys (dammit, where has she put them?) in the knowledge that, shit, I'm already late!

Hmmm, it's unlikely that our conscious approach will actually work, is it? The results only come when targeted in a subconscious environment.

It's this simple: if we do not learn to have better posture in a subconscious environment, then we do not learn to have better posture. Many of my students and the clients of their students claim to be taller as a result of using the AiM method. This is because they have moved from one awareness of posture (slumped, kyphotic and protracted) to another, more upright and effortless posture that they have achieved from working in a three-dimensional environment, following the five big rules and achieving a subconscious state of balance. Not only are they taller – they have less pain and far more potential than before. It is truly amazing and inspirational, it humbles me every time.

Let's not force change on our clients, but use movement to inspire change from within. Often in a movement session, you can feel things clicking back into place – triggering me, about five years ago, to nickname this work 'osteopathy in disguise', or body transformation. Movement allows the body to reorganise itself to experience the effortless motion I described earlier. So I'm not forcing change, the body is simply accessing it through the tool of movement.

If we do not learn to have better posture in a subconscious environment, then we do not learn to have better posture

WHAT THE FOOT?

→ NEUTRAL NONSENSE: YOU
CANNOT MOVE EFFICIENTLY
WHEN HOLDING ONTO
NEUTRAL SPINE

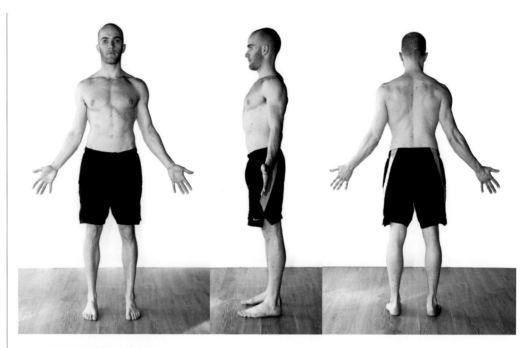

RANT #8: NEUTRAL SPINE

This is simple and I'll cover it more in big rule #2 later. Neutral as a concept or goal for training and rehabilitation is utter nonsense. It's impossible to move in a neutral position. Try it. Set yourself up: neutral spine, neutral pelvis, neutral shoulder girdle and neutral feet (if you can) and now take one single step. Whoah there! Try again. Notice how as soon as you even thought about moving you lost your neutral position. You can't hold it and move at the same time SO why bother?

Training and exercising in neutral is also a problem. It's a static concept that is safe and risk free when under load. Which is kind of true. EXCEPT that by not being able to move comfortably away from neutral,

back to neutral, through neutral and away again is a huge problem for your movement and your mobility, even in a load-bearing squat. You should know that neutral spine is a mere moment of time amidst the total array of movement possibility, even in a simple gait cycle and, if the truth be known, in a squat, too.

Neutral gives us an awareness of our optimal centre position, but has nothing to do with how our body wants to experience movement. It's a similar problem to rant #7. If I force neutral spine on you as opposed to encourage you to find that neutral point yourself — something I will call 'centre' throughout this book — then I am pouring effort into your system and stabilising you when what I want to be doing is liberating your body to be strong and mobile in a free-flowing environment.

RANT #9: KNEE OVER TOE (STABILITY OF ANY JOINT)

My penultimate rant is always the big one. Once again there is a dichotomy with the beliefs of the strength and conditioning world, and seems to bring together many of the previous eight rants I have just laid before you.

To keep your knee over second toe is to stabilise the knee and foot in a bid to maintain neutral foot and pelvis during a lift or movement. It's an attempt to keep the knee safe under load and the science for that is strong. YET it doesn't happen at all in movement and is even well documented.

I have a video here at **www.whatthefoot.co.uk/ kneeovertoe** that highlights how the foot, ankle and knee interact in movement, thus proving that to keep the knee over toe in lunge and squat patterns, not to mention keeping knee over toe as a sports–specific approach, makes absolutely no sense at all.

In a bid to make the knee safe, you are in actual fact making it weak for the longer term. At the same time you are eliminating the role of the human foot and ankle and are consequently omitting any possibility of a relationship between the foot, ankle and knee. Clearly, they are connected since the ankle (tibia, fibula and talus bones) connects directly through the long shaft of the tibia to the knee joint (tibial plateau, patella and femur). I have a feeling it might continue this journey up to the hip, don't you?

A safe knee is one that can freely move in accordance with the ankle. If the foot collapses the knee naturally moves towards the midline. If the

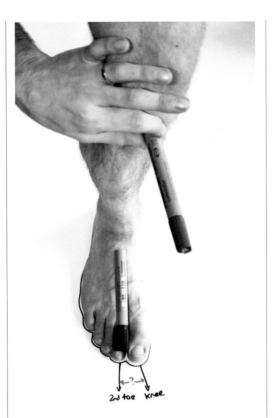

2nd toe knee

← IN STANCE POSTURE THE KNEE RARELY, IF EVER, SITS OVER SECOND TOE. TO DO SO WOULD REQUIRE A PERFECTLY CENTRED FOOT AND ANKLE

foot supinates strongly the knee naturally moves away from the midline. To have zero awareness of this motion, that is to say to not experience this movement in a controlled exercise environment (ie keeping knee over toe in exercise), is synonymous to making the knee strong in one position that it may well never get to experience in its everyday movements – since, thanks to poor foot posture, it rarely ever sits perfectly knee over toe. Like neutral spine, knee over toe is a mere moment in time (if you are lucky).

A safe knee is one that can freely move in accordance with the ankle. If the foot collapses the knee naturally moves towards the midline. If the foot supinates strongly the knee naturally moves away from the midline

WHAT THE FOOT?

→ A SPORTSPERSON IN ACTION WILL ALWAYS FIND THEMSELF BRINGING THE KNEE INSIDE SECOND TOE — NO MATTER HOW MUCH YOU COACH THEM NOT TO DO SO. SO WHY BOTHER?

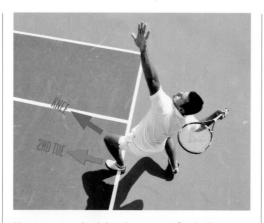

In my work with footballers and athletes, a rounded awareness of the relationship between the hip, knee, foot and ankle always leads to an improvement in performance and a return to the playing field. The knee is designed to move, and is not designed to be stable

It's my personal opinion that many a footballer and tennis player (read any athlete!) has suffered knee, ankle and groin problems as a direct result of squatting and lunging whilst purposefully, consciously, limiting the range of motion at the knee and ankle for fear of causing any damage and in favour of protecting the knee.

In my work with footballers and athletes, a rounded awareness of the relationship between the hip, knee, foot and ankle always leads to an improvement in performance and a return to the playing field. The knee is designed to move, and is not designed to be stable.

The last thing I will ever do is stabilise the knee, provide support to limit movement in the foot or limit natural movement in any exercise or rehabilitation approach. Like the avoidance of stretching, I have never had a problem with this and have always had rapid and long-term success. This goes for all and any joints in the body.

On that note, when a knee problem walks into my studio, I also have a strong suspicion that the problem is not in the knee, but in the relationship that the knee has with its surrounding structures.

COMFORT ZONE

To stabilise anything is to create a big fat comfort zone around it. We all feel powerful and mighty within any comfort zone we build around ourselves — that's why we build it, right? Until, that is, we are forced to venture outside of that comfort zone; into what might be called a 'dark zone' where we are unsure of ourselves and feel exposed and at risk.

DARK ZONE

I describe the end range of movement as a dark zone: somewhere the body doesn't like to go or daren't go for fear of something going wrong. Entering the dark zone is a bit like facing your fears, jumping into a room full of spiders, for example, and coming out alive, phobia free, a stronger and better person. You realise that you had nothing to worry about all along. Always ask yourself what's the worse that can happen. Enter the dark zone and you will always come out stronger, or hide away in your safe place and always remain limited in your potential. Growth and potential develop only when you step into the unknown and challenge yourself to do or to be better.

It's no different for the knee. When the knee is trained to be over the second toe, it generates its own comfort zone about that point — powerful and mighty! As the knee moves medially along with a pronation of the foot, it becomes exposed, at risk and unsure of itself. In the video above you will have noticed the range available to any knee in natural movement is so much bigger than this 'knee over toe' space. The comfort zone NEEDS to be as big as that whole range of movement, and not just down

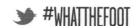

WHAT THE FOOT?

the midline. Imagine having newfound strength in those dark, never before visited spaces (both medial and lateral to the knee) and imagine the increase in strength you would naturally have in the 'knee over toe' space. The midpoint will always be stronger than the extreme ranges, and it is fair to say that the midpoint can only be as strong as its relative extremes.

Here now lies the problem with training knee over toe: at high speed, in a high-performance non-linear environment such as football, tennis or dancing, it is IMPOSSIBLE to keep the knee over second toe. In gait or walking, the knee is NEVER over second toe apart from a moment between pronation and supination. The good news is that muscles in the body are perfectly set up to allow, control and manage the medial position of the knee, AND all muscles need to frequently go there in the training, exercise and rehabilitation of the knee. The knee needs to visit its dark zone on a regular basis if you are to get strong in this position. And since virtually every step you take goes there anyway, whether you are walking or playing football, it is a good idea to focus on NOT keeping knee over toe when training for movement.

This idea is so ingrained in you, the reader, that we always, always arrive at a sticking point on the courses when this subject first comes up. But ask any AiM practitioner now and to them the idea of stabilising the knee is a joke. Why? Because the fewer knees they attempt to stabilise, the fewer knee problems they see. Mobility equals more and more healthy knees.

MECHANICAL ADVANTAGE

Once again, if you are squatting huge loads, it's not necessarily a good idea to let your knees and ankles

roll in! The mechanical advantageous position is clearly knee over toe because it creates a column over a rigid foot structure where the strength at this midline of movement is strong relative to the strength at the extremes.

However, watch any heavy lifter and you'll notice that when they get to the bottom of the squat they naturally, subconsciously, flatten the feet and bring the knees inside second toe in order to generate sufficient power to return back up to the rest position. They naturally break the 'knee over second toe' rule – even though their coach is bawling at them not to! Why? Because that is how the body is set up to work. Big rule #1 explains this phenomenon. If you are an S&C coach, one thing I might suggest to you is that if and when you see this happening, please don't try and coach it out of the athlete – it's the way the body works and we must respect that.

There is no way a footballer or tennis player, golfer or skier can keep their knee in this position full time, yet in the gym they are shit scared of venturing away from it, recognising it as a 'bad' position. Just remember, if it was bad, we wouldn't physically be able to go there, but we can and so we must teach the body to deal with it. In fact, if the body can do something, we must make sure we are capable of doing it and doing it well.

GET OUT OF YOUR COMFORT ZONE

Think of your body and posture as always being in a comfort zone, a place it knows well and is happy to exist, safe in the knowledge that nothing can go wrong. To make the most of this posture, it pays to visit the various dark zones of your body, explore the end ranges and take your joints and muscles to those 'unexplored' spaces.

WHAT THE FOOT?

If it hurts, don't go there, and if it doesn't hurt, go there frequently... Simple!

Encourage muscles to have no option but to contract, give joints the opportunity to experience a fuller range of motion,   and notice how your comfort zone and awareness of self will grow. When you wonder whether or not you should take your knee inside of the big toe, remember to ask yourself 'what's the worst that can happen'? Use an informed answer as opposed to embracing the fear that has been placed in your head around this discussion, based in old-school science.

One very simple rule: if it hurts, don't go there, and if it doesn't hurt, go there frequently. Ask yourself which muscles are perfectly set up to control this movement – you should be able to feel it.

No growth can occur within a comfort zone – your body cannot reach heights or opportunity beyond its imagination when governed by a comfort zone. Only by venturing out into the big wide world, challenging your comfort zone and entertaining dark spaces, facing your fears, can you recognise and face up to your present boundaries and restrictions. For once you go beyond them, you will make new boundaries, have new limitations and new fears, but you will have moved on and gained strength, rendering old boundaries part of your now comfortable territory.

WHERE DO THESE RANTS COME FROM?

Each rant has a common flavour: each one is hardwired into the brain of therapists and trainers the world over. Each rant sits on one side of the coin. In order to create an environment for amazing results to occur, simply oppose each and every one of these rants. Do the opposite and see if something new and amazing happens. There's

a list coming up on page 46 of possible to dos for you.

I know that you feel like you get amazing results now and that your clients are grateful and love you for your work and come back again and again. I used to think the same until I realised the huge escalation in my results using the five big rules, and the enormity of admiration from my clients and students hit another level, not to mention personal satisfaction.

When I talk about perceived centre later on in the book, remember this: you are currently in a perception of what works well for you and is normal for you and in that state you appear to be the best that you can be. It includes the best service you can offer and the highest knowledge you have attained. You should give yourself a pat on the back for this. Do it now.

Sadly, however, it is the case that when you increase your knowledge or change your awareness, that perception of yourself and your skills changes with you. Have you ever been on a course over a weekend and on Monday morning completely changed the way you work with someone? Of course you have. We all have. New skills are exciting and powerful, more powerful than what you did yesterday, simply because adding a new skill into your own pit of knowledge adds even more value to the skill itself... and to you! Looking at movement transforms your awareness in this way, enhances what works for you now and advances the service you offer.

This happens because to truly understand movement adds a whole new dimension to your

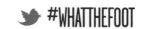

work. For instance, if you have only ever worked with someone on a couch, the shift in your approach will be 100% dramatic because it's 100% different to work with someone standing up and moving. They move differently upright to when they are on the couch by the way. It's not the same.

This is reflected in the two-sided coin model. I'd like to take a look at what this looks like in the industry today and what it could look like in the industry tomorrow.

You guessed it: the current industry focus is on the left-hand side of this coin.

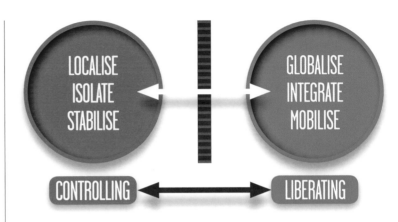

Localise
To localise something is to shine the laser on it – focusing the attention on a single structure, that area being part of the greater whole. In the example of the body, a localised treatment would focus the attention on a single structure, for example, the knee.

Isolate
Isolate is slightly different. When you isolate a joint, you exclusively focus your attention on the workings of one joint, forgetting all others. An example again would be to mobilise the knee or ankle without paying attention to the relationship that that knee or ankle has with surrounding joints and structures.

Stabilise
As discussed in the rants, to stabilise something has become a profound way of addressing the joint system. I see it more as a 'fear'-based approach in the majority of situations. To stabilise

a knee, ankle or low back carries the intention of protecting it despite the fact it ultimately exposes the structure to the risk of limited movement. We have misunderstood when and how stability is present in the body and, let's face it, not for the first time. We have all been sucker punched by a classic piece of marketing not unlike the 'fat kills' campaign, which dominates people's minds and nutritional programmes.

Whenever I tell a patient/client that I no longer want to focus on stability they all say the same: "I thought we needed a stable core?" When I ask why, they never have an answer for me... students, too.

I'll always reply with: "Oh, but we do need a stable core – we just need to generate it through mobility." All will become clear.

Controlling
It's a very Western philosophy to control the world around us to feel like we are in control of our life.

We have misunderstood when and how stability is present in the body

WHAT THE FOOT?

Focusing on pain, as we all tend to do, when it is present puts the nervous system into a fight/flight state and things head downhill rapidly

Isn't the irony that inside of us all there is a desire to be liberated or set free?

If you dig down deep to the core of people's highest values, most of them will end up saying "I want to be free!" Your body is no different – it needs liberating from the shackles of limitation and stabilisation in order to feel freedom and flow. On the current side of the coin, this, sadly, is not actually a possibility.

I'll give you an example of two ways of looking at the same thing and experiencing completely different outcomes. Try this:

- Take a moment to settle your mind and get into your body.
- Now I want you to pay attention to all the places in your body that have pain, any pain, the slightest sensation. Anything.
- Spend a moment focusing on that pain and become really aware of it.

Write down what and where you feel it; also take note of how it makes you feel.

_____

_____

_____

- Now retune into your body.
- This time pay attention to all the places in your body that have no pain, nothing at all, areas that feel clear, light and breezy.
- Spend a moment focusing on those areas and become really aware of it.

Write down what and where you feel it; also take note of how it makes you feel.

_____

_____

_____

_____

Done correctly, this should produce a very different feeling in your body and in your mind. More importantly, there will have been a subtle (or noticeable) change in your nervous system.

What you focus on expands – and, in this case, focusing on pain-free areas is nourishing for the nervous system and creates more of that. Expansion.

Focusing on pain, as we all tend to do, when it is present puts the nervous system into a fight/flight state and things head downhill rapidly.

May I suggest that we are really, really good at helping people focus on their pain in both the allopathic and therapy communities. Even though we have the patient's and client's best interest at heart. Focusing on the pain, minimising movement in a sore joint and stabilising (for fear of moving it too much) creates the second response in the nervous system – a fear-based one. We become attached to our pain, we focus on it, harness it and give it all the attention it needs to thrive and remain with us for years. Oh, and we must protect it, control it and manage it. How would you feel?

WHAT THE FOOT?

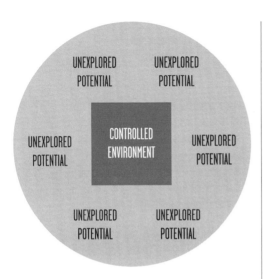

↑CONTROLLING THE MOTION OF A KNEE IS AKIN TO LOCKING IT DOWN AND MINIMISING ITS POTENTIAL. TEACH IT TO EXPLORE THE UNEXPLORED AREAS AND WATCH IT THRIVE

The circle above allows us to overcome that.

Globalise

Think of your local environs and then think of the globe. Imagine the globe in your hand. In order to have the largest possible impact, would you change the way your local community thinks, or would you change the way we think on a global scale to have even more significant and long-lasting change on the many smaller communities?

It's obvious isn't it? In that sense, movement is the globe and the knee is the local community. To focus on the body as a whole is to work at a higher logical level and have greater impact on the whole system. When I work with knee pain, for example, I rarely ever have to actually look

at the knee itself. I take a global perspective and the treatment filters down through a complete mobilisation of the physical and neurological structures.

Integrate

Again, slightly different. Integration is more about understanding the relationship between one joint and another. What is the knee doing when the ankle is doing x? No, it's bigger than that: what is the knee doing when the ankle is doing x, the hip is doing y, the big toe is doing z and the opposite shoulder is doing n?

Sounds a bit crazy and difficult to perceive, does it? Well, I have news for you: there are no stable joints in the human body when it is in motion. This means that we can plot every movement in relation to another movement at every other joint in the body in three dimensions of movement and in each phase of gait!

The good news is that you don't have to work this out for yourself as I have already done it for you!

I have mapped this fully in what I call the flow motion model and am now in a position to teach it to you so you can see it, feel it yourself and use it to eliminate pain and unleash new levels of performance in all of your clients.

So you have a choice: you can either choose to sit and work it all out for yourself or know deep down that I would truly love to help you fully understand it. If you are anything like me you'll feel the need to satisfy the geek within you that has an innate need to understand the human body at the highest level possible.

WHAT THE FOOT?

If you think the knee needs stabilising – go and do it; if you think the knee needs mobilising – go and do it

Integration is the one thing that the brain understands and is the one thing that you need to understand to work with the body at the highest level possible.

Integration is not something we can think about on the left-hand side of the coin. The problem is that most movement educators do tend to think about movement without integration and I like to think that that is where Anatomy in Motion is satisfyingly different.

Mobilise

I'm sure I've said it before and I'll say it again. Mobility is the one thing that the body must make use of if movement is to be possible. Mobility in all joints creates an awareness of what is possible in each and every joint, thus creating a safe awareness of movement potential about a mechanically advantageous point for the joint. We call it 'centre'. To know your centre is to be efficient, have flow, conserve energy and to be liberated from the shackles of limitation and stabilisation.

In shiatsu, they say your body is a river, ever flowing: this is only possible if there is motion. Stabilise a river and you create a dam – stagnant and limited in its intended potential.

RETURN TO THE RANTS
Is it worth briefly looking at what it would mean to oppose the rants?

Rant #1: Static stretching
Solution #1: Dynamic mobilisation
Rant #2: Separating eccentric and concentric actions
Solution #2: Marrying eccentric and concentric movements
Rant #3: Core stabilisation
Solution #3: Core mobility
Rant #4: One-dimensional training
Solution #4: Three-dimensional training and movement
Rant #5: Reciprocal inhibition
Solution #5: All muscles are synergists working for the same goal
Rant #6: Localised treatment
Solution #6: Integrated and globalised approach
Rant #7: Forced or conscious activation
Solution #7: Natural and free-flowing unconscious movement
Rant #8: Neutral spine
Solution #8: The spinal gyroscope
Rant #9: Knee over toe (stability of any joint)
Solution #9: Exploration of maximal movement per joint in an integrated environment

Now imagine that you understood how to use both worlds and thought processes and could freely access both in your daily work.

If you think the knee needs stabilising – go and do it; if you think the knee needs mobilising – go and do it.

At least you have the choice, whereas before, to stabilise was the only option. If nothing else, there is huge power in that, isn't there?

RANT #10

There is a 10th rant – of course there is – and I think it's this: it's the failure to accept the body as a closed, integrated and unpredictable entity.

In conventional therapy we are not taught to work with the body as a whole. Science breaks the body down into parts, into smaller and smaller pieces, and does its utmost to understand everything about each little piece of it. Has it helped? Yes, to a certain extent this has given us a therapy industry and we now know more than we could have hoped for back in the early days of scientific exploration into the human body. However, one thing is dramatically overlooked. It's that the human body is a closed system. It can not exchange any part of itself (other than heat or work/effort) with the external environment. All of its parts remain intact at all times, though may change the way these parts align or are used, to maintain energy conservation in the system. Each part being reliant on another to understand its own role means that all parts are interdependent and thus must experience change as a whole and not as individual units. My rant is simply this: the more we look deeply at the isolated aspects of human anatomy and the longer it takes to link all

this information back together to inform the body as a whole, the longer we run around like headless chickens looking for the answer, and being human beings, we naturally believe the answer lies in the smaller and smaller parts, so we dig deeper and deeper.

And yet right there in front of us is the beautiful human body, giving us answers to all the questions we've ever asked. It moves in a way that is perfect. Closed, reliant on all parts. Effective in its misgivings, too, ie even when it doesn't work well, it still gets the job done!

When the foot hits the ground a whole-body reaction occurs. When the foot hits the ground in a perceived dysfunctional way, the whole body reaction will be different – the way we walk will be different, the way we experience our body will be different – and I can bet that a whole host of reactionary changes occur on the smaller and deeper levels, too. My rant is not that isolated research on the parts of our system has been wholly embraced, but that research on whole-body motion has not been. There are a few scientists and researchers who have great interest in AiM and its work and yet the universities they are connected to fail to open doors for research to be carried out to try and prove some of what I am going to tell you. It's a two-sided coin problem where all research lives on the side of the coin that has led to each of the first nine rants.

It's highly likely that you've spent a serious amount of time learning the ins and outs of localised anatomy. So take some time to pull back a little, switch off the laser and shine a light bulb over the whole package, take note of it all, simultaneously, as we step into the five big rules of motion.

> *The more we look deeply at the isolated aspects of human anatomy and the longer it takes to link all this information back together to inform the body as a whole, the longer we run around like headless chickens looking for the answer*

CHAPTER 3:
THE FIVE BIG RULES OF MOTION

"It's not wise to violate rules until you know how to observe them." **T.S. Eliot (1888-1965)**

Not to be confused with Newton's laws of motion, these are my laws – Gary's big rules of human movement. The five BIG RULES that flip convention on its head and offer new ways of working and thinking about how the human body works. They are designed to reflect the side of the coin that our testing of dead people failed to bring into reality. In fact, it's what I created over the years as a direct result of working with people who were very much alive and experiencing instant change – I simply had to sit down and work out what is actually going on. Once again, this is good news, since you don't have to carry that burden. I really want to share it with you.

The five big rules are as follows:
● Muscles lengthen before they contract
● Joints ACT, muscles REACT
● Everything orbits around centre
● Perceived centre dictates movement, posture, pain and potential
● Perfection is hardwired and pre-installed

What I'm about to say is completely understandable and is the case with every course I teach: I bet for the anatomists out there, you struggled to even get past the first two! As discussed, this is because, traditionally, the lengthening (stretching) component

and the shortening (contraction) component of muscle have been separated. Quite simply, we stretch and we strengthen as two different things.

Also, when the muscle is stimulated through EMG the dead person's muscle contracts (shortens) and the bone subsequently reacts, creating a named action in the relative joint. Naturally, we have believed this to have been the case for years now. However, in movement-based anatomy it does not happen this way. What's important to recognise is that it can happen this way, but is not necessarily supposed to. The third big rule may appear a bit abstract, but all will become clear, whilst the fourth and fifth big rules simply state that our perception of normal may be far removed from the ideal and it is this state of 'normal' that influences our wellbeing. Normal is to thrive in the comfort zone even when pure potential resides in the dark spaces where most people dare not go. Are you ready for a trip down the rabbit hole of human anatomy on the flip side of this two-headed coin? I hope so...

The first caveat, I guess, is to remind you that we are discussing movement, not regular anatomy as we know it. In this case, since we are discussing all things on the flip side of that coin, it is my suggestion to you now, that you park what you know or what you have been told, somewhere out of the way (far out of reach) and we'll bring it back in later. Remember, it's both sides of the coin together that bring the most value to the human body. All of this information is simply an extension of what you already know, something to add in to your work and complement your already fantastic knowledge with. If you aren't sure about something I say, remember to add the words 'in motion' to the end of it – it's all relative to how we move and not to how we lay down or be still.

Scientific validation?

I think it's also quite important to raise a flag at this point and say that if you are looking for scientific validation throughout this book, I am not really offering it up to you. Most science exists on the left-hand side of the coin, as expressed in the previous chapter. Whilst I can see the validity of movement in the science that exists and relate it to my work, I personally place a higher value on the experience than I do the science. This may not win me any friends, but I don't really care about friends – I care about results and understanding! Often, when people throw science around in support of a particular method, it contradicts what I am doing, thereby invalidating the science in my mind, whilst further consolidating the belief in the person of the methodology they chose to use, effectively supporting their choice to remain in their own comfort zone. So I am here to challenge you in your thoughts, challenge the industry as it stands and challenge what science has to offer in the world of human movement as I see it. All of the rants in the previous chapter (with the exception of the 10th) are heavily supported by science, and yet their use in exercise and therapy terms frustrates the hell out of me because I can see another way that incorporates the science, but adds to it as well. I'm looking at the parts that the papers failed to pick up on as they chose to look for something in support of a knowledge that already existed.

Incidentally, with countless biomechanical papers concerning gait available, which provide the platform for our scientists to understand human movement, wouldn't it be a disaster if we could disprove the ancient theory it's based upon? The inverted pendulum, sagittal plane lever systems... That's the process the new study of human movement is undertaking. If we rewrite the old by bringing in the new, then how we work, how we understand the body and the results that are possible can change. Once we used smoke signals, now we use iPads... We are stuck in a crazy comfort zone that may not even have an ounce of truth in it.

I make no apology for that. I know that how I work with people is effective. I know, equally, that my students get the same results that I have been able to. I know it's repeatable, it's a transferable skill and is seemingly what the body wants to experience for that rapid and long-term shift. So I probably won't take a step into the expected view of the world as, in truth, it doesn't do that much for me. I'm interested in change, huge shifts from one state to another and even quantum leaps! There are a few references that I shall make where I feel it necessary or simply rude not to, yet, in the main, the ideas in this book are born from my experience and are my determination of what is going on in the world of anatomy. I'm simply sharing what the body does and highlighting some truths in that. Most likely, it's the case that what the body really does and what you think it does are not the same thing. Again, I only say that because it shows up on every course I have ever taught and virtually every initial contact I have with a therapist. There is so much more to know and explore... so shall we do it?

> *I know that how I work with people is effective. I know, equally, that my students get the same results that I have been able to. I know it's repeatable, it's a transferable skill and is seemingly what the body wants to experience for that rapid and long-term shift*

BIG RULE #1: MUSCLES LENGTHEN BEFORE THEY CONTRACT

In the outback of Australia, kids are taught to deal with a snake by stretching it from head to tail, fully lengthening the muscles of the reptile to put it in a state of survival, to defend itself through the action of contraction, reducing the snake from a state of attack to a state of submission. The further apart the head and the tail get pulled, the stronger the snake must contract its whole self to protect itself. Muscle lengthening, or eccentric movement, is essentially a defensive motion to control the separation of two moving parts. The stronger the snake is in this motion, the less the risk of injury and threat. The weaker the snake is in this motion, the greater the risk of injury. It also happens to be the way the muscle develops most potential and most power, so as the two parts move away from each other the muscle is generating a response from which a powerful contraction must take place:
i) to control the movement
ii) to develop forwards motion

Maximum contraction potential

How is it that activating the glutes can relax the hip flexor, but activating the hip flexor deactivates the glutes?

I have a simple question for you: From which position does a hip flexor have maximum contraction potential? A neutral position or an extended position?

I have seen many clients who have been advised to stretch hip flexors and strengthen glutes. What happens here is that the patient is asked to move his hip from neutral into an extended position against resistance and/or to hold a static stretch in extension.

Excellent therapists and trainers among you will know that an extended, abducted and externally rotated hip results in maximum glute contraction and a subsequent hip flexor stretch. However, for both the glute and the hip flexor, which have an obvious synergistic relationship, this is only half of the story. The missing component to hip extension is hip flexion, to bring both sides of the coin together. It is as simple as that for big rule #1.

A professional footballer whose training and therapy programmes were locked tight into the concentric world – shortening muscles from a neutral position and pushing harder and harder to get greater results – was wasting his talent on the therapy bench and not on the pitch, since every time he took to the training ground his body broke down again. Shortening the quads, shortening the glutes, shortening the hip flexors, stretching the hamstrings, stretching the calves and shortening the abdominals and adductors in the vain hope of a positive outcome! The approach was not working, yet was tried over and over again with the expectation of it one day finally working. This, as Einstein put it, is the definition of insanity – except when your steadfast beliefs allow you to think that what you are doing is actually worthwhile and has value for the client. In this case it was neither worthwhile or valuable to him or his team, but no changes to the approach looked like being made! Ever!

I introduced big rule #1 to Bradley Orr, then of QPR Football Club, privately, over a period of two sessions and the results were incredible. He went

WHAT THE FOOT?

from not playing through the first part of the season to featuring in over 90% of games that season, uninjured and fully involved in a Championship winning team, something he could easily have missed out on had he not altered the approach to his therapy.

He had this to say: **"One minute I have no chance of playing at the weekend, next minute I'm pain free and feeling confident about the game with no concern of injury. That to me is priceless.**

"I know I will use Gary's method for the rest of my career, he has helped me over the phone, in person and via video – I've never known anything else help me stay on top of my physical form like this. There is no bigger compliment I could pay."

Let's take a look at this first principle of human movement then: muscles lengthen before they contract – always!

Concentric first = compensation and limitation

What EMG testing and research tells us is only part of the story – a tiny part in fact. In motion, pure fluid and efficient movement experiences no contraction of any muscle prior to its lengthening. If that happens, you are actually witnessing faulty or inhibited movement patterns – your body in compensation.

Conventional anatomy has got lost somewhere along the way – and when you read this you'll probably recognise that you already know this and wonder why you haven't applied it in such a way before!

Thanks to EMG testing we discovered that a body laying on a table will contract its muscles

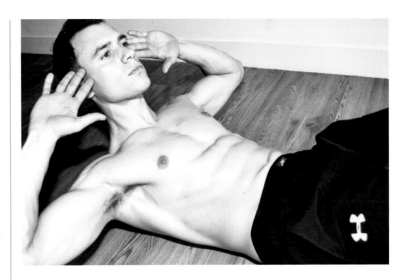

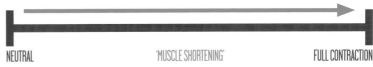

NEUTRAL   'MUSCLE SHORTENING'   FULL CONTRACTION

from a neutral position to one of maximum shortening, where it cannot contract anymore (see above illustration).

However, in natural uninhibited movement this never happens, and yet our exercise industry is fully based around the concept of muscle shortening. It makes us strong, gives us big muscles and is aesthetically pleasing.

It also happens to be a huge factor in posture, pain and potential.

The bit that has been forgotten about is the fact that a muscle can shorten, not just from the neutral midpoint, but from any given point on the

Our exercise industry is fully based around the concept of muscle shortening. It makes us strong, gives us big muscles and is aesthetically pleasing

WHAT THE FOOT?

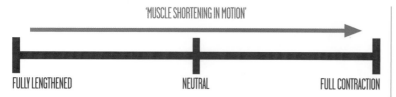

'MUSCLE SHORTENING IN MOTION'

FULLY LENGTHENED   **NEUTRAL**   **FULL CONTRACTION**

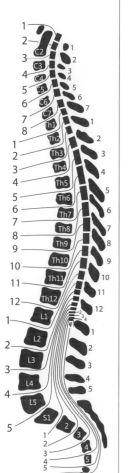

contraction curve. In fact, the maximum amount of shortening or contraction that can take place is from a muscle's most lengthened position.

What's that? Yes, a muscle has maximum contraction potential when it is contracted from a pre-lengthened position (see above).

It's still shortening, but from a lengthened position. The difference now is that the muscle is passing through neutral, as opposed to starting at neutral, and contracting over twice the length than before.

Which reminds me...

Neutral nonsense
The concept of the neutral spine, as I mentioned in rant #8, is utter nonsense. And, for that matter, so is the concept of any neutrality in the body whatsoever from the feet, to the pelvis, through to the shoulder girdle. To be in neutral is a futile exercise. It's a great reference point for us to assess how far we are away from it, but it's a useless concept for us to try and attain. The neutral point is a mere moment in time – something we visit for a fleeting moment, if at all, during movement.

What is neutral spine?
Neutral spine is set where all vertebral joints of the spine are in neutral, relative to the bone above and

below it. It's how the spine should look, as in the diagram to the left.

A neutral foot sits midway between flat-footed and high arched, where all the bones line up perfectly to form the three arches. A neutral pelvis sits in perfect balance, not tilted or rotated, and likewise for a neutral shoulder girdle.

In this position you'd probably look like a guard stood outside Buckingham Palace, erect, tall and proud.

However, as soon as you intend to move away from this position, you are no longer in neutral spine. EVERYTHING has changed.

Human movement is certainly not a topic for radio! Some visual sequences need to be seen to appreciate this, but my point so far is that to aim to be in neutral full time is nonsense, whilst to have the awareness to move away from it and back to it again and again is one of the keys to fulfilling your physical potential.

You see, we have hung our hat on the idea that neutral is vital, yet in everyday life this neutral position for the lucky few is a tiny moment in time as our huge frames simply wink at it on the way by. For the remaining many they won't even get anywhere near neutral as they have literally no awareness of where this point is at all.

Let me explain something: you are one of the many if you have bad posture, rounded shoulders, pelvic anomalies and flat, high-arched or turned-out feet. I am now talking about upwards of 90% of you – including you fitness and therapy professionals!

Most therapists and trainers are obsessed with teaching this position to their clients and focus on being strong in this position. What you probably haven't considered is that your client may not even be able to hit this position in their daily movement and therefore are simply throwing money at fresh air in a vacuum.

You may have gathered that I am not a fan of the word 'neutral'. I think as a concept it is hugely flawed and have chosen to describe it in another way. I call it 'centre'.

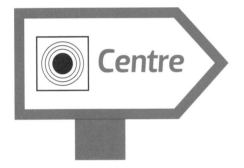

All you need is a signpost.

Centre

Centre is the midpoint of all things. This means that in order to know where centre is we have to experience the full possibilities of what lies beyond that centre point. If I ask you to pinpoint the middle of a circle that isn't even on the paper yet, then you are going to struggle. This is how your poor body feels! It has no awareness of where its outer limits lie and therefore no concept of where its maximal and optimal centre point lies. At this point you can still think of centre as neutral if you like – it's neutral, but within a specified three-dimensional range.

So here's the thing: in isolation, all muscles have the capacity to stretch to one side of this centre point and contract all the way back to the other. It's called range or range of motion. Conventionally, we separate the two ends of this spectrum and treat them as two separate things, with the outcome being to either stretch or shorten muscles. In therapy we stretch at end range and in exercise we shorten to end range from neutral, yet in your daily movement – and by that I simply mean walking, getting out of a chair, picking your child up, etc – you actually access both in one smooth motion, from one end range to another, passing through the centre point.

My simple view on this is to create movements (call them exercises if you will) and treat patients to incorporate all of this... Because it's what the body does!

Range

The only way to fully appreciate the range that a muscle has, is to find its maximum range of motion. If your body has no awareness of this maximum range of motion then it will have no awareness of where its centre point is and that dream of achieving your peak potential dwindles away daily.

Fully shortening muscles and stretching muscles is not the solution either. Our brain can only experience the range that it has available to it, even if there can physically be more. When we introduce more range into the system, in an integrated environment, it will naturally begin to access it in daily life, making what was once limited in range now freely accessible.

We get the body and brain to achieve this by lengthening muscles first – taking a muscle to end range to give a muscle its full contraction potential. The elastic property of muscle means

The only way to fully appreciate the range that a muscle has, is to find its maximum range of motion. If your body has no awareness of this maximum range of motion then it will have no awareness of where its centre point is and that dream of achieving your peak potential dwindles away daily

we can use a catapult as a simple way of describing muscle motion.

The catapult effect

Pick up that catapult and ask yourself: "How am I going to project this little rock across the field?" Answer: by lengthening the elastic as much as I can.

Pull the elastic halfway back and you'll see a pathetic response from the rock as it drops out of the sky by your toes! Pull it all the way back and the rock will effortlessly glide across the field.

Your hip flexors on the front of your hip are designed to bring your leg forward in swing, not from underneath you, but from behind you. It flexes most from its most extended position. The further you can pull that leg back (by placing the other leg forward), the more fluid the forward motion of the hip flexor (and leg) will be. Just like the catapult!

No option but to contract

When the hip is fully extended (and by fully, I mean you can't extend it any more) then the muscles that are required to flex that hip have no option but to contract and bring the hip forwards in flexion.

To give a muscle no option but to contract you have to put it in its most lengthened position. Not just in one dimension, but in all three dimensions in which that muscle functions. In this way, you can kick-start a dormant and inactive muscle in seconds.

Let me be clear, if the muscle still has range in extension available to it, then there remains both an option to flex or extend – to give it no option but to contract into flexion would require full extension being taken up.

Many, if not all, of your clients have 'sleepy' glutes. Glutes that have little or no involvement in the day-to-day running of things. The brain is simply bypassing the glutes to avoid the effort required in using them. Currently, the conventional side of the coin suggests activating the glutes through concentric contraction, thus isolating the muscle and actively, consciously, shortening the muscle from a neutral position to its maximum shortened range.

On the movement side of the coin, we simply look at how the body works. Since muscles lengthen before they contract in motion, the lengthening has a specific purpose, to create an environment for the muscle contraction to take place.

Dormant muscle activation

Taking any muscle, reviewing how it contracts and putting it into the opposite joint actions will easily activate any dormant muscle, such as the glutes. The glutes are easy: they extend, abduct and externally rotate the hip. If I place the dormant glute maximally into a flexed, adducted and internally rotated position, then can you see how that muscle now has no option but to contract into extension, abduction and external rotation?

EXTENSION   'OPTIONS AVAILABLE TO THE HIP FLEXOR (SHORTEN OR NOT)'   FLEXION

FULLY LENGTHENED   'NO OPTION BUT FOR HIP FLEXOR TO CONTRACT'   FULL CONTRACTION

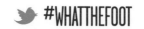

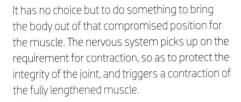
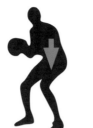
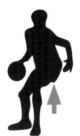
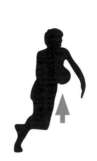
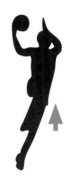

It has no choice but to do something to bring the body out of that compromised position for the muscle. The nervous system picks up on the requirement for contraction, so as to protect the integrity of the joint, and triggers a contraction of the fully lengthened muscle.

In essence, what I am saying is the glute extends the hip from a flexed position, abducts the hip from an adducted position and externally rotates the hip from an internally rotated position.

Once you can do this for all muscles in the body, you will witness a fascinating reaction in the bodies and the faces of your clients.

Right now, we are still looking at muscles in isolation. When we are upright, on our feet and in motion, we have to take into account the whole body. We cannot move one part of it without moving other parts of it – in truth, without moving all of it.

It is a fully integrated system where once we move anything we actually move everything. Does this mean that all muscles are lengthening at once in motion? No – only those that are required to decelerate skeletal movement. Does this mean that all muscles contract from their pre-lengthened state then? Yes. Any concentric contraction in the body requires too much effort and is normally a compensatory response to faulty movement patterns.

Which is why I wonder and rant at the concept of training the body with concentric movements only. The body doesn't work that way. Having said that, if you can think clearly around this concept, try pre-lengthening the muscles you want to train before you do a concentric contraction and you will be combining the concentric–eccentric metronome of movement, which has a far greater specificity for movement. So again, you can simply add a dimension to your concentric workouts. How would you lengthen your pec as much as possible before contracting it?

Load to explode

When you jump up, which way do you go first? Down. When you throw a ball forwards, which way do you take the ball first? Backwards. In both cases, the muscles for jumping up and throwing a ball forwards are pre-lengthened or 'loaded' before the action can successfully be executed.

The bigger the load or lengthening, the greater the muscular contraction and the more explosive the force that the muscles involved will execute – even if one of the muscles in the chain was previously dormant. It would now have no option but to get involved and what was previously a weak link in the chain now contributes evenly to the whole movement, reducing the pressure on the other muscles to compensate for its failings and creating a more even and balanced interaction throughout the muscle chain.

I have successfully trained sports coaches and NLP practitioners, who have little or no knowledge of anatomy, who are able to execute this work and get results where others (trained therapists) haven't, simply by following this big rule: muscles lengthen

When you jump up, which way do you go first? Down. When you throw a ball forwards, which way do you take the ball first? Backwards. In both cases, the muscles for jumping up and throwing a ball forwards are pre-lengthened or 'loaded' before the action can successfully be executed

before they contract. If your sport involves movement, which I know it does, then apply this to yourself and notice the transformation in your mobility, strength, balance, speed and power.

Still, it takes a little bit more to understand this process better, which is why there remain four more big rules. Suffice for now to say that all muscles move more freely and optimally when: a) they come from a lengthened position; b) they get to experience full range; c) are given no option but to contract; and d) journey right through that centre point and beyond.

IN SUMMARY

▶ **Muscles lengthen before they contract.**
▶ **The further you draw back a catapult the greater the potential for the object to fly far and true.**
▶ **Maximum contraction occurs from a maximally lengthened position.**
▶ **Muscles thrive on whole ranges.**
▶ **Muscles work on a continuum of two extremes with a midpoint.**
▶ **Muscles are at their most relaxed at this midpoint.**
▶ **Muscles can equally access both ranges from this midpoint, rendering awareness of this midpoint indicative of potential.**
▶ **Importantly, muscles thrive on the awareness of whole ranges to know where that midpoint is.**
▶ **A muscle's ability to be effective relies on:**
➡ **all other muscles being effective;**
➡ **an effective joint system; and**
➡ **whole-body awareness of centre**

BIG RULE #2: JOINTS ACT, MUSCLES REACT

Jennifer, who had been diagnosed with scoliosis after seeing a chiropractor, with pain referring down her arm accompanied by significant pain in her shoulder, contacted me for help.

Her X-ray showed she had significant scoliosis in her thoracic spine as it snaked up between her ribs on either side of the spine.

The reason she was experiencing pain in the shoulder and arm was a direct reaction to her skeletal (spinal) alignment. Her muscles were being pulled all over the place and the nervous system was compromised by her posture. The impact on her gait and physical movement was very clear to see, and the foot scan assessment made it very clear to see how she was walking and standing with the omission of very obvious and basic patterns.

The movements I decided to use encouraged her body to access movements and physical spaces it had not been for years. As joints moved into previously unobtainable spaces, there naturally had to follow a direct influence on her muscle and nervous system. You can see how she weight bears predominantly on her left leg thanks to the scoliosis posture. What if her scoliosis meant she could not weight bear on the right foot? What if I teach her to weight bear on the right foot in both stance and walking? Her muscles and joints have learnt to favour her left side over her right, so if I can convince them otherwise... Since the positions that her joints did not regularly have access to succinctly fit into one of the key movement patterns taught by AiM, it meant that Jennifer had one key exercise to perform that would reinstate the old patterns

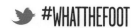

of movement and impact directly on the spinal alignment. Our first session changed everything for her. The closer to centre she gets, the straighter her spine has to be...

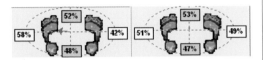

⬆ IMAGE TO SHOW BEFORE AND AFTER WEIGHT SHIFT AND PRESSURE PERCENTAGES (BEFORE: LEFT, AFTER: RIGHT)

...and so it was, she began weight bearing through her right side in stance and in walking and the feeling through her body was one of liberation.

Jennifer is not alone. Had I focused on changing muscle tone, either manually or using a foam roll, I could not have brought long-term relief to her because the skeletal patterning of how she walks and moves on a day-to-day basis would not be challenged, and the joint system that influences the muscle system hierarchically in movement would remain the dominant force, forever returning the muscle length to its painful resting state and allowing the posture and skeletal alignment to remain unchanged and unchallenged.

Let's discuss this new phenomenon at length: joints ACT, muscles REACT.

Reaction
We discovered, in the last section, that there is a dual role of muscles. They have a simple role to play:

lengthen – shorten – lengthen – shorten – lengthen – shorten

That's what muscles do ALL day (even when you are asleep and breathing!). To place and hold them in neutral is ultimately to limit their experience. Especially when we talk about big rule #2.

All this muscle action that we talk about is interesting, but it changes again, or, at least, we can add dimensions to all of the above by understanding this next statement:

All muscles do all day long is REACT.

The simple term 'muscle action', again coined through the history of anatomical research, is once again flawed and it would serve you better to consider the muscle reaction as opposed to the muscle action.

How so?
Without being too technical here, there is a situation where muscles are not contracting first to create movement, but are reacting to the position of the skeleton in space, such as discussed in big rule #1 with regards to the glutes. When we are walking, the foot hits the ground and a reaction occurs whereby the foot rocks from heel to toe and drives the body forward. Sounds simple, and yet when we slow this movement right down we begin to notice that it's not muscles that are guiding the movement of the skeleton, but this thing called gravity and our reaction to that in relation to the ground.

Everybody has heard of pronation, right? It's where the foot flattens and is apparently the thing that we want to stop happening (more on this later). What's interesting is that in movement there would appear to be no muscles that actually serve to pronate the foot.
None.

Had I focused on changing muscle tone, either manually or using a foam roll, I could not have brought long-term relief to her because the skeletal patterning of how she walks and moves on a day-to-day basis would not be challenged

WHAT THE FOOT?

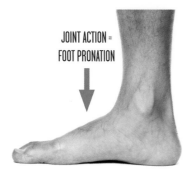

JOINT ACTION =
FOOT PRONATION

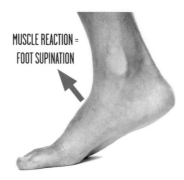

MUSCLE REACTION =
FOOT SUPINATION

Everybody has heard of pronation, right? It's where the foot flattens and is apparently the thing that we want to stop happening (more on this later). What's interesting is that in movement there would appear to be no muscles that actually serve to pronate the foot

As the foot enters the ground, it is simply gravity and the clever articulation of the bones of the foot that allow the foot itself to collapse towards the ground and away from its restful, peaceful centre point.

It does this for one reason and one reason only – to stimulate the muscles of supination in the foot and extension in the rest of the body, via a lengthening process, to force a reaction and pull the foot out of its flattened state and propel the body onto its toes and forward into the next step.

The bones of the foot move first and the muscles react to that movement. It could be said that the 'opposite' muscles react to slow down the rate at which the foot is collapsing. It's a kind of safety mechanism that taps into the body's innate desire for survival. Is that what this could all be about?

Now, as I said earlier, if one thing moves, then everything moves. So when the foot enters into this pronation collapse, the knee is mobilised, the hip joint adapts, pelvic alignment changes, the spine moves away from its revered neutral (already?) and the shoulder girdle is forced into motion as well since

it is attached to the ribcage, which is connected to the spine.

Utter chaos... but very clearly, joints move first and the muscle and fascial system manages that movement.

If there is a group of muscles set up to slow down the movement of the foot to generate desired movement then it goes without saying that there are muscles perfectly in place to slow down the movements of the other skeletal body parts I just mentioned as well.

Which muscles decelerate the knee, pelvic and spinal motions and react to these movements in such a way that they kick-start perfect full-body motion into the next stride?

Put another way: which muscles are given no option but to contract in order to control the movement of everything?

It could be said that rule #2 should be 'Joints REACT, muscles REACT', since joints react to each other's motion and to the ground/gravity relationship as well. In which case, our whole body is simply reacting to the world around us. Thus, it is how well you react that dictates how well you move and ultimately how easy your life is.

We are looking to create a perfect balance between the outside world and our internal environment. When external influences are equal to the internal influences, then we reside in a state of perfect balance: centre.

Each reactive movement in the body creates a lengthened state in the muscles, which are set up to

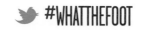 #WHATTHEFOOT

defend that joint's journey away from centre. When a muscle has allowed suitable motion in the system to generate enough force to propel the system forward, then it shall stop the joint from going one way eccentrically (away from centre) and contract it back in the other direction concentrically (towards centre and beyond). This point is known in AiM terminology as the 'point of zero motion' – where eccentric stops and concentric starts – otherwise known as the isometric point of movement.

This tick tock mechanism goes on all day from one point of zero motion to another, and not just when you are walking, running or jumping either. It literally happens all day long! It never stops. Remember I said earlier that we are never ever static? That simply means that movement is ever present in our physical system.

As the joint approaches end range, a muscle must contract to control that movement and bring it back towards centre. As the skeleton as a whole moves away from the centre point, a whole group of muscles will react to control that global movement and bring it back towards centre.

Inhibition

The tighter a muscle is, the less distance it will allow a joint to travel and the more another joint will have to travel to accomplish the overall goals of the body and brain. Now we have entered the realm of compensatory movement. This can only occur when the body is performing suboptimally.

In the same vein, any joint inhibition or limitation means that muscles cannot experience their full range of motion and will start to lose power and force output. It also means that the joints next to it

or further away in the system are not receiving the appropriate neurological messages. Things spiral slowly downwards into reduced performance, and potential for pain arises as your body downgrades itself and performs suboptimally.

When it comes to movement therapy, we have to look at range of movement in the joints when in motion to determine what impact they will have on the muscle and neurological system. In the same way that bones, joints and muscles are all connected, so we must accept that the nervous system is, too, and any movement we do or make affects the communication around the body to the brain and vice versa.

Good healthy promotion of movement relaxes muscles, promotes excellent joint integrity and stimulates the nervous system. Any movement inhibitions cause the opposite effect and that's not good in anybody's book – particularly this one.

Like many things in this world, the body is a three-dimensional entity. The majority of joints move in three dimensions – not all of them; joints do what they can to facilitate global movement. This means that there is a single centre for a multitude of movements. In order to now have some awareness around that point, the body has to experience full three-dimensional movement patterning.

Again, in movement, everything is moving all at once and so it's possible to plot the movement of any joint by seeing what dimension(s) it's travelling in and coupling it with another joint. In this way we can determine if a joint in the foot is moving in tune and appropriately with another body part – no matter how far away from the foot it is. When all

Good healthy promotion of movement relaxes muscles, promotes excellent joint integrity and stimulates the nervous system. Any movement inhibitions cause the opposite effect and that's not good in anybody's book – particularly this one

WHAT THE FOOT?

It's not the muscles' fault that you can't stand up straight – they are actually making sure you don't stand up with even worse posture than you do now!

body parts move in tune with each other perfectly, then we have optimised movement, created a balanced environment, enhanced posture and set a base from which peak performance is now a possibility.

Static posture

Next time you think about poor posture and that the muscles are pulling the skeleton into that position, think again and recognise that the muscles have actually organised themselves so as to manage that posture, prevent it from slipping further away and are putting their own functionality at risk in the name of function. It's not the muscles' fault that you can't stand up straight – they are actually making sure you don't stand up with even worse posture than you do now! Your first thought is that some muscles are tight, some are weak, some are inhibited, others facilitated and you want to stretch them, strengthen them, massage and foam roll them... But it's not the muscles' fault – the weakness, tightness and inhibitedness comes from the skeletal position and the resultant reaction taking place in the muscles.

I know this because of big rules 1 and 2 combined – muscles are lengthening and shortening to accommodate the skeletal position and not acting to distort the skeleton, as we appear to currently think. I also know this because in skeletal alignment, once we have taught the body to find centre, and posture is restored, muscle lengths change back to normal in seconds.

WTF?

Full understanding of our second big rule actually means you can be successful with the human body

without ever knowing muscles in detail, their names and their origins and insertions (which are all just labels anyway). You can simply move and mobilise the skeleton itself into end ranges or dark zones to challenge its comfort zone, giving the muscles no option but to fire up, manage the system and begin to work as a global unit to optimise overall movement potential of the body. This creates a new comfort zone and a quantum leap in your potential will have taken place.

From old to new in a matter of minutes...
(not months).

For those of you who think fascia instead of muscle and how the usage of fascia supercedes muscle, I have to say that this still applies. You would be right to think that fascia is a higher logical level than muscle, but wrong to think that fascia influences the skeleton IN MOTION. It's the same principle here: joints ACT, fascia REACTS. More on fascia later...

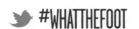

IN SUMMARY

▶ The length of a muscle depends wholly on the organisation of the joint system.

▶ The organisation of the joint system depends wholly on its relationship with the ground, both in static and dynamic posture.

▶ Muscles like on-off-on-off-on-off and their ability to do so relies on motion and freedom in all joints.

▶ To hold a muscle still in a stretch is to neglect the role of the joint in the function of that muscle.

▶ To mobilise a joint in isolation is to neglect the role of the muscle chain connected to that joint.

▶ Muscle weakness, tightness and inhibition comes from skeletal position and joint motion – the reaction taking place in the muscles leads to the inhibition.

▶ Muscles and joints must communicate and work together if effortless motion is to be attained.

▶ In isolation, muscles seem to carry huge importance. From a whole or total standpoint, it's clear they form a partnership with the joints and are employed, in motion, to react to the movement in the joints. Joints ACT, muscles REACT.

BIG RULE #3: EVERYTHING ORBITS AROUND CENTRE

John was injured playing football 20 years ago, when he ripped the left side of his ribcage/serratus anterior at high speed and in his words "blew out four lumbar discs at the same time". He spent a year in hospital and has been in agony ever since. When he saw that he had over 70% of his bodyweight through his right foot, he instantly and unconsciously understood why his body had hurt him so much over the past 15 years and wondered why nobody else had bothered to investigate this.

Two sessions later, when he saw that his body weight was now evenly distributed 50% /50% through both feet, he instantly understood this third big rule and how it related to him miraculously being pain free for the first time in 20 years. He could both see and feel the transformation in his body.

This case study is laid out in full on page 106.

Centre is a key concept for understanding movement and it's no surprise we find this big rule in the middle of the five. What comes before and after it depends wholly on getting to grips with this big rule. It's the little twist in your understanding of centre and the change in your thought processes that challenges everything you thought you knew about anatomy.

There is a centre in everything

If you are a sports coach, and haven't considered the impact of the centre of mass on your athletes and how they manage that centre of mass, then you are missing a large part of effective sports-specific training and coaching.

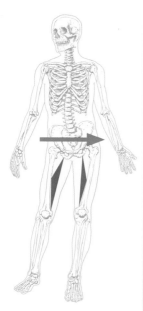

↑ ADAPTATION IN THE SKELETON CHANGES LENGTH TENSION IN SURROUNDING SOFT TISSUE. HERE THE RIGHT ADDUCTOR LENGTHENS TO DECELERATE THE PELVIC SHIFT AND THE HAMSTRING LENGTHENS TO DECELERATE ANTERIOR TILT. IN A FIXED STATE THESE BECOME LONG AND TIGHT

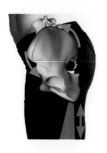

Everything, and I mean everything, has a centre, including your emotions. If you are never happy or sad, then it becomes impossible to describe what emotion you are experiencing in that context. Yet someone who has experienced the full range of happiness and sadness would be able to pinpoint exactly where they stand on that spectrum at any given time.

Everything in your body has a centre, too. Biomechanically, we are talking about the centre of mass. Your centre of mass is an aggregate of all the bones, muscles and mass that you carry in your body. Each individual bone, joint and muscle has its own centre point, be it the centre of mass of an individual bone, a midpoint in joint range or a balanced relationship between two or more muscles that causes a relaxed and balanced state around a joint.

Anomalies in these alignments of centre are what create the postures we currently perceive as problematic.

Vladimir Janda created a way of looking at the human body that discusses muscle tone adaptations in opposite muscle groups when a relaxed and balanced state between joints and muscles is not present. He called them 'upper' and 'lower' cross syndromes.

He suggested that muscles are either phasic or tonic with some crossover (ie some muscles could be both). Phasic means set long and tonic means set short. Both of these descriptions suggest (to me) that the muscle itself would be 'off-centre' – too short (tonic) or too long (phasic). He would use words like inhibited, tight, long and weak to describe

them. Most commonly I hear muscles described as either a) short and tight or b) long and weak. For me, this grouping of terms is not specific enough and it's clear, to me at least, that different patterns can appear when assessing the body in movement.

The normal grouping of terms in this case is for a muscle to be 'long and weak' or 'short and tight'. Every time a student catches me saying the phrase 'long and tight' together I get the following response: "Sorry, did you say long and tight?"

Yes, I did...

I have noticed on a regular basis that there are different reasons for this. A muscle can be tight both when:

a) it is in a lengthened state and where stretching would ordinarily be advised; and
b) it's in a shortened state and in a permanent state of contractile effort.

For a muscle that is tight and in a lengthened state, I have a small bit of advice: **there is absolutely no point in stretching a muscle that is already long!**

There may be grounds to stretch the muscle mentioned in point b), but I would prefer to locate the reason for this hyper-contraction.

Beside the fact that I have little or no faith in the static stretch, I am forever presented with people who have been told to stretch the wrong muscles!

Rightly so, a therapist might recommend a stretch of the tight muscle in an isolated context where some pain is present. That is to say, that when a

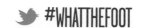

muscle appears tight in this way, to stretch it seems an obvious go-to. However, only in a whole-body context, where a comparison is made between one side and the other and is cross-referenced with overall postural alignment, can we judge why that muscle is tight in the first place and whether it is tight because it is a) long or b) short.

It can be both. Refer back to the horse's head analogy (page 27). A long hamstring, as in the image, will be tight if its resting state is long, due to a fixed anterior tilt of the pelvis.

An adductor, as in the image above, will be tight if its resting state is long, due to the pelvis shifting laterally away from the leg in question: it is literally fighting, in reaction to the skeletal alignment, to pull the body back towards its midpoint and a state of balance. It is this sensation of fighting that leads to the tightness — pelvis shifting one way and the muscle pulling back. It's a tug of war. A stalemate.

Once again, I hear people inform me that they need to stretch this 'long and tight' adductor, and once again the problem is that the prescribing practitioner has not noticed that it is the overall shift of the skeleton that has caused the tension in that adductor. Stretching will not help; only an overall realignment will take the perpetual stretch out of this adductor and allow it to rest once and for all. This type of realignment is what I call 'finding centre' — teaching the body to naturally optimise the alignment of its own centre of mass.

Finding centre
Since there is a midpoint to everything, there must be a point in the human body that we can call centre. As I will explain, centre is a complex arrangement of our centre of mass, our base of support and a perception of the way we are, including how and why we hold our posture in the way we do. The key to centre is not knowing where it is, but to be able to encourage the body to find it on a consistent and ongoing basis.

When working with the body, rather than stretching an already lengthened muscle or treating the joint in isolation, I prefer to teach the joint in question to find its own centre.

To do this I target all of the muscles responsible for managing the joint in question and ask them to decelerate that joint in all three dimensions in order to develop a full experience of what movement that joint should be able to successfully achieve. When both the muscles and the joints have full range available, the joint determines its centre point from where it can freely access all available ranges, compromising none, and each muscle falls into a state of balance — because they have to.

The reason the original muscle was tight in the first place is purely down to the fact that the whole system was moving in an adapted manner and the muscle in question had no option but to remain in a lengthened state.

So, stretch the muscle? Or target the system as a whole?

To 'find centre', target all of the muscles responsible for managing the joint in question and ask them to decelerate that joint in all three dimensions in order to develop a full experience of what movement that joint should be able to successfully achieve

TARGETING THE SYSTEM AS A WHOLE

"Doctor, Doctor, I've been stretching my tight left hip flexor, but I still have pain."
"Stretch the other one then."

Stretching the other one is an unconventional, yet vital, thought process since the painful left hip flexor you are stretching is long, relative to the opposite hip flexor! It is the muscle that is fixed in an over-long state that is where the pain is felt. By 'stretching' the other one, say through eccentric mobilisation of the right hip, we can change the relationship that the pelvis and both hip joints have with both hip flexors. To move towards balance, or find centre, is to lengthen the short muscle and shorten the long (problematic) one, thus relieving the pain.

This is not an unusual conversation to be heard in my clinic. Except the doctor part, of course – which is a shame because if I was, more people would probably listen to me!

Targeting the system as a whole has a natural and holistic feel about it, doesn't it? That's the kind of thing that happens in acupuncture and reflexology or shiatsu and other weird and wonderful therapies. Not what you really want for your running injury though, is it?

You feel like you want the sore muscle massaged, despite the fact it could have been triggered by the uneven movements in your feet. You want the local area to be treated even though the cause most likely lay elsewhere in the system. In movement therapy we work on the higher logical levels as discussed before. This is where the environment is treated as opposed to the specific problem.

Stretching the muscle in question is the lower logical level, where we hope it impacts on the greater system; treating the whole body in its natural reactive state is the higher logical level where change happens in the system as a whole, thus eliminating the pain or inhibition that arose as a result of the overall failing of the body in this adapted, reactive state.

If we take a look at modern therapy, it's fair to say that most people visit their therapist to be treated on the couch. Using movement can act as a useful extension to this environment. Let's assume there is a problem with the joints in the feet and the client has a hip problem. The desire to examine and treat the hip is massive. "What's going on in there?" leads to digging around the hip and making certain assumptions about the hip itself. Half an hour's treatment later and the pain will have eased, you feel better, you hand over your money and you are out the door. Engaged in the action of walking, however, step after step, the untreated problematic joint in the foot continues its poor movement and re-stimulates the negative reaction in the whole body, which slowly stresses the hip again... thankfully your therapist has already booked you in for next week!

I often find it amusing to wonder what the client thinks when they come with pain in their back and I start fiddling with their feet!

Teaching the whole system to react better to the outside world is a far more natural way of working, and it would appear to be what the body and the

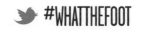

brain wants. To bring the whole body into balance, or to find centre, is a key process for getting people out of pain.

The extension to your work that movement offers, is the one where you treat the hip in question, ease the discomfort and then mobilise the hip and the foot so they learn to speak to each other again, re-communicating effective movement and contributing better to the success of the system. When you do this, you have the best of both worlds. You are accessing both sides of the coin, working at a higher logical level and it's natural to see better, high-quality, rapid and longer-lasting results.

Balance

Balance is a harmonious relationship between two polar opposites. In physical terms, it's the alignment of the whole system. Your aim as body workers is to create this relaxed and balanced state between all joints and all muscles in the body to achieve exceptional awareness of your centre and eliminate any short, long, tight, weak combinations or tendencies. You want all muscles to be at their optimal vital length. I access this information by studying your centre of mass — a wonderful indicator of where your whole body is in space.

Mass management

Another phrase I use for balance, which tends to lead us to balancing on one leg or our hands, is 'mass management'.

Balance on one leg is only possible when we have our centres in alignment. A handstand only becomes possible when we have our centres in alignment. Gait is only possible when we learn to manage our mass, mobilise it from one foot to the other and have our centres in alignment. The centres I am talking about are our centre of mass, centre of gravity and base of support.

Centre of mass

When we calculate the average centre of mass of all bones in the body, we come to the overall centre of mass of the human body. It lies approximately in the region of the naval, an inch or so below the belly button, and often collides directly with the L4/L5 inter-vertebral joint in the spine.

L4/L5? Isn't that the most common site for back pain in the world?

Imagine if this were purely down to the fact that our centre of mass was slightly to one side or out of optimal alignment, forcing pressure onto a spinal disc. What if you taught a client to manage their centre of mass better earlier in the therapy process and you could have avoided that problem? Just what if?

For instance, imagine your centre of mass (represented by the white dot in the images to the right) has shifted towards your right-hand side — you would carry more weight through your right foot than your left foot. Consider the consequences of all muscles attached to this poorly aligned system, each muscle reacting to the new postural bias. Which one do you want to stretch now?

Consider what position the joints or individual structures, such as the pelvis and the spine, would be in as a result of the reaction to the position of the centre of mass? Perhaps you can feel it in your own body or see it in somebody else's?

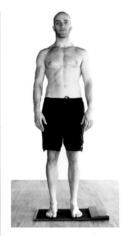
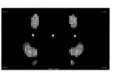
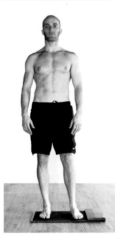
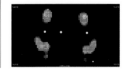

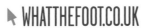

Alignment and mass management takes place when centre of gravity and centre of mass are in line with each other and comfortably within the base of support

Before fully understanding this concept of mass and what it means for the upright individual, we need to first have a look at the 'base of support'.

Base of support

When you stand upright, your base of support can be described as the area around both feet and the area in between your feet (represented by the blue line in the images below).

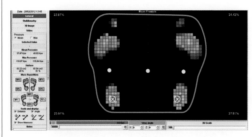

As we take our feet apart the base gets wider, and as we bring them together the base gets narrower. As we shift our weight fully onto one leg the base of support now includes the area of the foot in contact with the ground only.

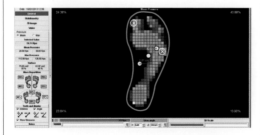

If we draw a vertical line down from our centre of mass onto the floor and call it our centre of gravity, it should lie roughly in the centre of our base of support (whether we are on one leg or two). We can be more accurate in this definition, but for now that is unnecessary.

What's interesting is the relationship between the base of support and the centre of gravity, and ultimately the centre of mass. The very fact I can stand upright at all is based on the relationship between these three things; not core stability, not neutral spine, not posture: since, if that were the case, judging by the state of the world's cores, spines and postures, we'd all be crawling around like vermin!

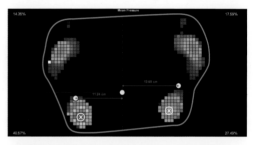

⬆ BASE OF SUPPORT AFFECTED BY ONE FOOT SLIGHTLY FORWARD.
BASE OF SUPPORT AFFECTED BY TURNED-OUT FEET ⬇

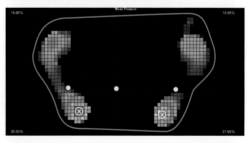

Alignment and mass management takes place when centre of gravity and centre of mass are in line with each other and comfortably within the base of support.

When my centre of gravity lies within my base of support I stand upright. This goes for standing on one leg or two. When my centre of gravity shifts outside my base of support, one of two things must happen:

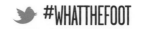

a) *I have to adapt my stance in order to remain upright; or*
b) *I will fall over.*

Once again, movement not being a topic for radio, you can refer to this link to see this in action: **www.whatthefoot.co.uk/baseofsupport**

On closer inspection, it is the moment when my centre of mass passes over the boundary of the base of support that everything must change. Everything has to change or I end up on my ass! When the brain and the ego kick in to realise the possibility of a) experiencing pain or b) looking a fool, you can bet bottom dollar that something has to change! At AiM we encourage the use of force plates for foot scanning as a way of assessing information about your centre of mass and its alignment within the base of support. The foot scan has the capacity to measure the movement of your centre of mass, which, for me, added new dimensions to the way I work with the body.

Challenge and support

Doctor John F Demartini, author of *The Breakthrough Experience*, claims that optimal growth occurs on the border of both support and challenge. Most of us felt challenged or supported through our childhood, for example – this sets a pattern for who we are in our future lives. If you spent your life growing up being challenged or in a challenging environment, you'll grow up 'hard' – another way of looking at this might be independent of others' support. Most likely you'd grow up harder or less dependent than someone who was raised in a fully supported, protected environment. You'd grow up 'soft' in comparison, or perhaps very dependent – 'wrapped in cotton wool' springs to mind.

Demartini also suggests that if you feel challenged in life, support will always be present, and advises you look for it to bring balance to any given situation. Likewise, when life feels well supported and easy, challenges naturally present themselves, so as to stimulate your opportunity for advancement or growth. His main point is that there is always a sense of balance, even when we perceive that there is not.

The base of support of the human can either be challenged or not challenged.

To stabilise skeletal structures by teaching the concept of neutral or following the core stability model is one way of NOT challenging the base of support. This is where we strengthen the body without experiencing movement towards the borders or perimeters of our base of support.

To mobilise the body over the base of support and take a tour of the perimeters of the base is the exact opposite. Movement allows the body, and therefore the centre of mass, to explore the boundary dictated by the base of support, enhancing our awareness of it.

Optimal growth and advancement in your physical prowess always occurs when your experience of the base of support is challenged. Remember that to challenge the body to increase the awareness of the support it has built around it and running through it, is to increase the potential for that body to stand on its own two feet.

In a modern therapeutic approach, support and/or stability is the focus, but where is the challenge? If the challenge is lacking, our opportunity for balance diminishes.

Increasing the awareness of the base of support is to increase the potential for the body to stand on its own two feet

WHAT THE FOOT?

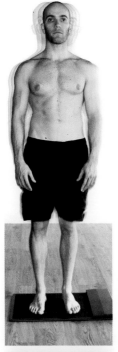

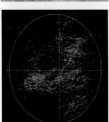

↑ EACH DOT REPRESENTS A NEW POSITION OF THE CENTRE OF MASS. EACH LINE REPRESENTS THE DIRECTION IT WAS TRAVELLING IN AT THE TIME. THIS SCAN WAS TAKEN OVER A PERIOD OF 10 SECONDS

This concept of mobility provides the opposite environment, the environment we want – an unbalanced framework for us to work in – one that mimics the natural movement of the human being, one that is set up for us to learn and develop within and one that we have accessed since birth and the early days of learning to stand up.

We can't actually stand still!

On even closer inspection, our centre of mass is never, ever, still. It's zipping about in a random fashion as displayed in the image on the left. This diagram is known as 'stabilometry' and is received from the foot scan software, which measures the movement of the centre of mass over a period of time.

There is no order to the movement of the centre of mass. It is completely unpredictable.

The centre of mass has its own base of support, if you like. It's measurable and I have seen it measure anything between $0.2cm^2$ and $5.5cm^2$ over a measurement period of 10 seconds. Over longer periods this number tends to get higher!

It seems inconceivable that this second person's centre of mass was moving over this amount of space, doesn't it? WHEN HE WAS ATTEMPTING TO STAND STILL!

The person who proudly holds the $0.2cm^2$ record, by the way, is an ex-athlete who had had stability drummed into her for years. Congratulations for being so stable? On the contrary, upon further investigation, her bodily movement and her aches, pains and problems were rife and yet eased when introduced to greater access to mobility and range.

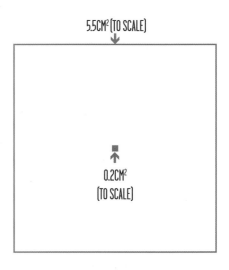

5.5CM² (TO SCALE)

0.2CM²
(TO SCALE)

This is the case whenever we see such small amounts of motion in the centre of mass.

Does that mean that $5.5cm^2$ then is the healthier specimen of the two? NO! He was experiencing way too much movement in his body and this was accompanied with his own problems and symptoms. In fact, what we found was, when testing over a period of 10 seconds, the measurement of stabilometry always returned to approximately $0.8cm^2$ or $0.9cm^2$, leading me to believe that this could be a normalised 'centre' or optimal amount of movement in the centre of mass for the system to be effortless.

Looking at the image again, there is never a moment of peace in the system. It's always moving. Our centre of mass, which lies just below the naval and is aligned with your L4/L5 vertebrae, is always, always moving. It never stops – ever.

Note that even at $0.8cm^2$ there remains movement in the system, thus there is always motion, always

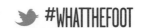

joint action and always muscular reaction – even in quiet standing.

This can mean only one thing: the human body is inherently unstable. Put in simpler terms, we cannot stand still and, in fact, we are anything but stable! I hope you don't mind if I suggest something...

Why, if this is the case, do we continue to strive so much for stability? Especially in our core, where the centre of mass lies, which can never be still in the first place? Come on, industry – now is the time to finally wake up!

My third big rule states that 'everything orbits around centre' - where the centre of mass goes, the whole body must follow.

More accurately is that there are certain patterns and ways in which the body does this.

With both feet on the floor, mobilise your mass, to the right, to the left, forwards, backwards, on the diagonals. Notice that there are huge changes to the way you stand. Your foot positions change, pronating and supinating; your spinal position changes, laterally flexing, rotating; your pelvic alignment changes with tilts and shifts. Now imagine you are stuck in one of these positions, with your centre of mass stuck over one leg or, worse, one heel.

What would be the impact on whole-body posture?

It is so easy to assess a client as wonky, poorly aligned or in need of some orthotics. Take your client's postural stance and exaggerate it. Exaggerate these stance positions a little – flexing more here and adducting more there. Now start

to feel things stretching. You are exaggerating in your body what your client is feeling consistently. Exaggerate your own posture and notice that stretch you have been doing - that you always need to do. Could it simply be a result of your centre of mass being off-centre? Can you feel it in your body?

Postural sway

It's highly likely that you are off-centre, by the way, since to carry your weight 50%/50% on both feet is uncommon. Again, the foot scan measures left to right weight distribution between both feet. If I'm right in my calculations, the chance of being 50%/50% is 1/100. It also measures fore and aft weight distribution – weight in forefeet or heels – and splits the base of support into four quadrants to break this all down. Ideally, there should be 25% weight in each quadrant. This is actually impossible to achieve since if we cannot be still, neither can the numbers. Regardless, the numbers and the position of the centre of mass do give us a strong indicator of how the body is standing and the overall impact on the body as a whole.

When we stand still, everything is already in motion. Biomechanically it is called postural sway. When we walk, everything is further set into motion. Movement gets bigger (more exaggerated) when we walk. Walking is a sequence of two feet on the ground, followed by one foot on the ground, followed by two feet on the ground. When there are two feet in contact there is a base of support that encompasses both feet, and when there is one foot down, that foot has its own base of support, too. The centre of mass always lies directly above the base of support, as discussed previously, and thus dictates the global position of the body when walking. Effectively, one foot passes the centre of gravity to the other and its

We are anything but stable

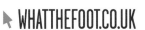

WHAT THE FOOT?

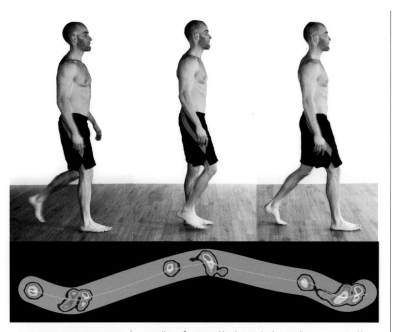

↑ ONE FOOT PASSES THE CENTRE OF GRAVITY TO THE OTHER AND ITS MEDIUM FOR TRAVEL IS THROUGH THE PATHWAY CREATED BY THE BASE OF SUPPORT

medium for travel is through the pathway created by the base of support.

Bear in mind the centre of mass lies above the centre of the pelvis. When the centre of mass moves, the whole pelvis goes with it. Can you, then, picture the pelvic movement through space? It would have to swing from one side of the body to the other, from above the single leg on one side to above the single leg on the other side and pass through the midline in between. The impact on the spine would be the same. My very simple point to make here is that there is no neutral in motion.

But there is a centre — many centres as it would happen — and our success in movement is relative to how well each structure passes through its own centre, moves away from it and returns back to it and beyond.

SOFT TISSUE REACTION TO INSTABILITY

This brings me onto muscular reaction in this unstable environment. Clearly, there is no order to the movement in the centre of mass — it appears to be random — which simply means that there can be no order to the movement of the skeleton either.

Quiet standing is not just unstable — it's utter chaos!

What holds it all together? What prevents the centre of mass from wandering too close to the border of its base of support?

It's obvious, isn't it? The muscles and fascia, of course.

Here we could bring fascial theory and myofascial lines into play. Simply put, these are a series of muscles which combine together to make straps of connective tissue that wrap continuously around the whole body.

With the rise in fascial awareness thanks to people like Thomas Myers, Phil Beech and Robert Schleip, it has become a dominant thought process that the notion of muscle is dead.

Personally, I still add huge value to the muscle, its attachments and the angles of force they produce. I do, however, agree that the concept of assessing and judging a muscle in isolation is dead — but not that the muscle is of no significance, ie dead, since it still forms an integral part of the whole system.

Fascial science is fascinating. No hard surfaces in the body are in contact or are able to make contact with other hard surfaces in the body, thanks to the fascial web that binds and envelopes everything.

Your bones, muscle cells, nerves, tendons, ligaments and organs are all wrapped up in fascia. Essentially one large fascial bag with hundreds of pockets, containing everything from muscles and bones to nerves and internal organs. I'm no expert on fascia, so I'll leave that to Tom Myers et al – but I am rather fascinated with how fascia contributes to movement or rather how movement contributes to fascial integrity.

Whether we choose to look at lines of fascia or choose to look at how muscles appear to operate in groups relative to any given movement, it's clear that there is a much bigger role that soft tissue plays in movement, on this side of the coin.

Deceleration

I have discussed how muscles act as a response to movement of the skeleton; they react to joint motion so as to slow movement down and return it back towards centre using an eccentric load of the appropriate muscle. That's on a micro level, looking at one joint and one muscle.

We then can look again at the same joint and recognise that a whole group of muscles are acting upon the movement of any single joint and working together to control that movement.

Technically, deceleration of any joint is accompanied by eccentric muscular contraction – not just by an individual muscle, but groups of muscle that have formed a relationship with the joint in question. To explain that more clearly we have to look at the contraction direction of muscle fibres.

For a particular muscle the fibres will always contract in the same direction. A muscle action, as we know, when contracting, has the effect of drawing two bones towards each other. This is known as a 'concentric' contraction – muscle fibres shortening under load.

An 'eccentric' contraction is when muscle fibres are lengthening under load to manage two bones that are moving away from each other. Interestingly, the direction of contractile force in the muscle is the same as in a concentric contraction. This is the same action, generally, that is what is stated in the anatomy books. However, in an eccentric contraction, the muscle action will be opposite to the motion in the joint that is being slowed down, ie a muscle will contract to flex a joint in extension and slow it down.

As long as the bones are moving apart at a greater speed than the muscle can contract, then the muscle will enter a lengthened state. The muscle uses its contraction action (opposing the movement in the joint) to slow down the movement of the bones, thus reducing the joint angle, moment by moment, until it finally wins the battle and brings the motion to a stop (the isometric point of zero motion). The muscle continues its contraction to initiate motion of the joint and bring the bones back towards centre – a relaxed length and position for both muscle and joint.

Think of it like this: in the diagram of the woman and the dog (page 72), as the dog moves away quickly and the woman tries to stop him, there is a period of time where the dog is moving away faster than the power required to stop him from moving. The force exerted on the dog is in the opposite direction to that in which the dog is walking. In this sense, the woman represents an isolated muscle that is required for the specific job of slowing the animal down. When the force of the woman equals the speed of the dog, the

A muscle will contract to flex a joint that is moving into extension

⬇ MUSCLE FIBRES ALWAYS CONTRACT IN THE SAME DIRECTION. WHAT CHANGES IS THE DIRECTION THE BONES TRAVEL IN. THIS DICTATES WHETHER THE MUSCLE SHORTENS CONCENTRICALLY OR LENGTHENS ECCENTRICALLY

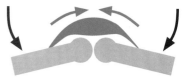

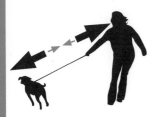

When the force of the woman equals the speed of the dog, the dog will come to a stop. For muscles (woman and lead) and bones (dog) it is the same

dog will come to a stop. For muscles (woman and lead) and bones (dog) it is the same.

The better the woman is at controlling the dog, the more freedom she can allow him. If the woman is a bit too eager, forever pulling back on the dog, the freedom is taken away from the little fella and the woman gets exhausted from unnecessary overexertion.

It's exactly the same for muscles: just as the woman manages the freedom of the dog, so the muscles appear to manage the freedom and flow of the body. Muscles that react too quickly limit and inhibit joint range, and muscles that don't react at all allow for too much range and inhibition in the body.

As mentioned earlier, any change in a muscle's role away from its optimal centre point means too much or too little range in a given joint, and the whole body must adapt to this environment, allowing for compensation anywhere and everywhere throughout the whole system.

If you have pain, this is happening to you, now. Muscles are long or short, overactive or dormant, and the skeletal postural balance is compromised.

If we look down from above in quiet standing, we can see how muscles are set up with the purpose of decelerating *any* movement of the centre of mass away from its optimal centre position. This is shown in the image on page 73 and described below.

As I lean forwards into my hip flexors, the hip flexors slow down that movement and contract to push me back. If I move perfectly out to the left, my left glute medius and ilio-tibial band (ITB) begins

to decelerate the motion, coupled with my right adductor, and together they work (contract) to pull me back.

Hopefully you can see how, as my centre of mass travels around my base of support, the muscles of the pelvis are directly influenced. In an altered posture-based stance – say, fixed forwards and right in my stance – you might notice how the right tensor fascia latae (TFL) muscle is positioned ideally to decelerate, control and manage that movement, but if posture is fixed in this position, i.e. persistently being leaned into, the TFL will adopt a lengthened, weakened and tightened state.

If the TFL appears inhibited in its functionality during a couch-based assessment, would you recognise that a particular cause of that might be how the client stands, relative to the central mass alignment of the whole body?

It's unlikely...

Global deceleration
With that in mind, we can look on a global level now, which is not just one joint or structure, but all joints and structures that make up the whole skeleton, and take a look at the whole muscle system that straps it into place, enabling us to hold together this thing called centre (or what we perceive as being our centre).

If every joint in the body has a multitude of muscles attached to it, then many muscles are required to work together to control or manage the movement in that joint. Each muscle has to play a part in the success of that joint. If one joint isn't successful then no joints in the body get the opportunity to be successful. If one muscle proves ineffective, then all muscles will be

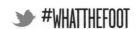

forced to behave differently due to altered joint angles and forces.

Therefore, it is absolutely essential to be watching over the whole body – to ensure efficient movement at all joints and in all muscles – if we are to have a positive outcome in somebody's pain or pursuit of peak performance.

Perhaps that is the ultimate role of soft tissue? To watch over the whole body, ensuring efficient movement at all joints and in all muscles as it goes about its day-to-day business.

Muscle management

If we look at the whole body, it's not crazy to accept that the big muscles in the body are on the outside of the body, under the skin and outside of the bone.

We have already paid attention to the fact that we can't stand still and have mentioned that the centre of mass can be measured and its motion revealed. Providing the centre of gravity remains inside the base of support we remain upright, so what is it that keeps the centre of gravity inside the base of support? Soft tissue: muscles, muscle chains or fascia – whatever you want to call it.

In fact, what's interesting (to me at least) is that muscles do not claim to be anything. That's our human prerogative, to give them names, labels and describe their actions and influence them in the way we believe to be right.

The muscle, however, simply does what is asked of it by the nervous system and does things that perhaps we had never considered before. They can be crazy things these muscles!

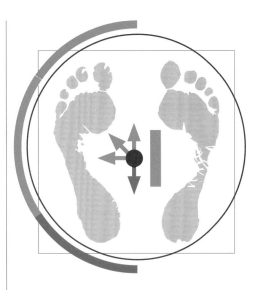

As the pelvis moves forward into the hip flexor, the hip flexor is loaded.

As the pelvis moves forward and left into the TFL, the TFL is loaded.

As the pelvis moves sideways and into the glute medius, the glute medius is loaded. Simultaneously, the opposite adductor loads as well.

As the pelvis moves backwards and to the left into the glute complex, the gluteus maximus and hamstrings are loaded.

In quiet standing, for example, the skeleton is attempting to minimise the amount of motion with which it orbits around the centre of mass. It cannot stop that – since movement is ever present in the system – but it can allow for too much or too little, which causes problems.

Firstly, I want you to consider fainting. Have you ever fainted or seen someone faint? The muscle system simply loses its awareness and fails to control the body from falling, and the only thing required to decelerate it is the floor racing toward it. Ouch!

When we are alert and have awareness present in our muscle system, the same movement of the skeleton is initiated and the body moves to a state of falling for a very, very, very brief moment. Then the muscle reacts. Skeleton first, muscles second. Joints ACT, muscles REACT.

↑ MUSCLES SERVE TO STABILISE MOVEMENTS AWAY FROM THE CENTRE

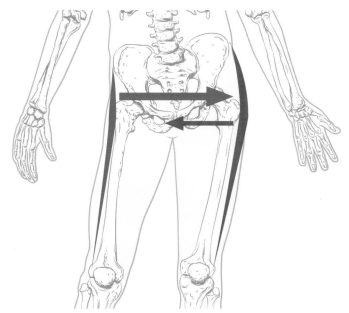

↑ THE SKELETON LEANS INTO THE LATERAL MUSCLE FIBRES (GREEN) WHICH DECELERATE THE MOVEMENT OF THE PELVIS AND CONTRACT TO PROPEL THE PELVIS BACK ACROSS THE BODY WHERE THE OPPOSITE SET OF MUSCLES (RED) WAIT FOR THEIR TURN TO REPEAT THE ACTION ON THE OTHER SIDE

As the skeleton leans into the muscle system, there occurs a natural lengthening of the muscles into which the body leans (see again diagram above). I often visualise them as trampolines, receiving a moving object, slowing it down and returning it from whence it came. For example, as my pelvis moves sideways into the trampoline (glute medius /ITB, etc), it stretches and expands and propels me back to the other side, where fortunately (or by design?) there is another trampoline-like muscle (opposite glute medius /ITB) waiting to receive the pelvis as it passes through centre.

It pays to consider whole-body muscle chains or fascial systems. Whichever direction the centre of mass moves in, it drives the skeleton to move with it in that same direction. There are muscles and muscle groups that run

the length of the whole body that are actually designed to slow that particular movement down.

Since Thomas Myers' Anatomy Trains book is so popular, I will use his fascial lines images to summarise how global muscle chains could lend themselves to control this motion of the centre of mass:

- When the skeleton, via the pelvis, falls forward, it is the superficial front line (SFL) that contributes to decelerating or managing the mass, lengthening and contracting to return the body back to centre or a position of ease.

- When the skeleton, via the pelvis, falls backward, it is the superficial back line (SBL) that contributes to decelerating or managing the mass, lengthening and contracting to return the body back to centre or a position of ease.

- When the skeleton, via the pelvis, falls sideways – it is both the lateral line (LL) and the deep front line (DFL) on the opposing side that contributes to decelerating or managing the mass, lengthening and contracting to return the body back to centre or a position of ease.

- With any rotation of the mass and the ensuing structures, it would be the transverse line (TL) that contributes to decelerating or managing the mass, lengthening and contracting to return the body back to centre or a position of ease.

- Should the pelvis fall on a forward diagonal, combinations of the SFL, LL, DFL and TL react to decelerate or manage the mass and return the body back to centre or a position of ease.

Apologies for repetition, but hopefully that concept lands more easily with you as a result of that.

As I said earlier, the further away from centre your centre of gravity goes, the more work your muscles

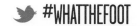

WHAT THE FOOT?

have to do to bring it back into alignment. If the centre of gravity approaches the perimeter of the base of support, there becomes a risk of falling over and so the muscles must work harder to prevent that from happening. In the fainting scenario, the centre of gravity literally 'passed out' of the base of support and no reaction took place to prevent the fall.

One other possible situation is that the centre of gravity physically moves outside of the base of support so quickly that the whole system must react by changing foot position to bring the centre of gravity back inside the new base of support.

In fact, walking is exactly like this... In walking, theoretically, the pelvis should be allowed to fall forwards beyond the toes and reacts to avoid a potential fall by placing one foot forward, thus taking a step and creating a new base of support.

To be stable in both static and dynamic environments there requires a strong awareness of mobility within a defined area that we want to be stable. All mobility takes place around the most efficient centre point or, more accurately, what the brain perceives to be the most efficient centre point (which will be discussed in big rule #4).

Creating stability at the centre point, i.e. in and around the neutral positions we discussed earlier, is akin to not developing movement at all, limiting joint range, teaching muscle to react too early to a movement, and limits movement in the whole skeleton.

Creating stability in a mobile environment allows for natural exploration of joint range, eccentric, isometric and concentric muscle reaction to take place, and gives freedom of movement in the skeleton.

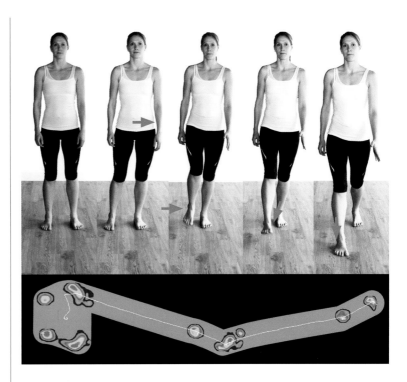

Stability is ultimately learnt by encouraging mobility in the system. Remember where the isometric contraction of muscle takes place? In the moment between the eccentric lengthening and the concentric shortening of the muscle, which is reacting primarily to the joint motion.

Remember the small square of 0.2cm²? This was the stable person, stiff, limited in range with awkward compensatory gait.

Remember the larger square of 5.5cm²? This was the wobbly person, stiff, limited in range with awkward compensatory gait.

↑ NOTICE HOW THE CENTRE OF MASS SHIFTS TO WITHIN THE BASE OF SUPPORT OF THE STANCE FOOT AS THE OTHER LEG IS LIFTED OFF THE GROUND TO TAKE A STEP

WHAT THE FOOT?

Stiffness arises in two forms, I believe: stiff short muscles and stiff long muscles

Stiffness arises in two forms, I believe: stiff short muscles and stiff long muscles.

Stiff long muscles being the head scratcher — no point giving them a stretch as they're already long! The thing to recognise is that a long stiff muscle will be found where skeletal alignment is compromised and the muscle has lengthened without having the force, strength, awareness or reason to bring the body back towards alignment.

An obvious example being where spinal kyphosis lengthens muscles of the thoracic spine. The muscles are not receiving sufficient stimulus from the skeletal system to encourage a contraction to bring the spine into extension and out of kyphosis.

Long stiff muscles spend all of their time attempting to both slow down further movement away from centre whilst contracting to bring the joint or a set of joints back to centre. The problem is they can't because the alignment of the whole system won't allow it. The brain doesn't want more kyphosis, nor does it know how (given all the parameters) to have less kyphosis — thus the body finds itself in its most optimal and perfectly functional state, for now. More on this in big rule #4. Needless to say, I hope, stiffness in any individual muscle is not a localised muscle problem; it's a systemic problem.

Once again, long stiff muscles are not muscles to stretch — more, they require a certain stimulation or to be given no option but to contract back to a more optimal and shorter length than they are used to.

Inhibition

Inhibited is a word used when discussing a muscle and its functional capacity. Ironically, muscle is inhibited when it is not optimal as the following charts show.

Force output or potential of a muscle reduces when:
- a muscle is too long or too short; and
- a joint's range is too much or too little

Force output or potential of a muscle is optimised when:
- muscle length is balanced in all three dimensions; and
- a joint's range is balanced in all three dimensions

For instance, we have maximum joint range, and therefore maximum force output potential of muscle, when the joint is at its optimum ROM. In the chart below this is shown at ROM[1], where optimum joint range equates to maximum force output at F^1. As we move along the curve, either increasing or decreasing joint range away from optimum, notice that the potential force output has to decrease down towards F^2.

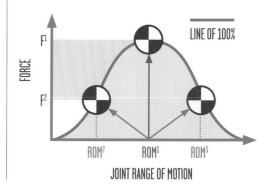

WHAT THE FOOT?

- ROM[2] represents a decrease in force output with less joint range available.
- ROM[3] represents a decrease in force output with a greater range available to the joint.
- Clearly, both represent a decrease in force output since any movement away from centre naturally leads to inhibition.

Likewise in terms of muscle: since joints ACT and muscles REACT, there is a natural carry over to the effectiveness of muscle length, too. Since F[1] is equal to optimum joint range of motion at the top of the bell curve, so it must be equal to optimum muscle length for that joint, too.

Any reduction in force output relative to joint range changes will see a natural adaptation in muscle length to either increase or shorten, relative to its role in the particular joint and the inhibition of the joint. In either case, muscle length changes result in reduced force output of the muscle AND the joint.

- L[2] represents a decrease in force output due to muscle shortening.
- L[3] represents a decrease in force output due to muscle lengthening.

- Clearly, both represent a decrease in force output since any length adaptation of muscle away from its natural resting length contributes to inhibition.

In both of these cases, the bell curve itself is known as the line of 100% – this is where I teach that **the body is 100% functional all of the time** – an explanation awaits over the next few pages, but for now, know that I interpret the body to be the way it is to support and contribute to your function as opposed to oppose it – it's functional 100% of the time. No exceptions.

So both the stable person and the wobbly person suffer in their bodies since this small factor of mobility in the centre of mass isn't optimally being managed by the muscle system. One has wandered one way up the bell curve, and the other has wandered the opposite way along the bell curve. Both still function and get on with life, but not as well as they could if their functionality were to be optimised.

Postural and dynamic stability arises in a fully mobile environment. It arises only with a full experience of where one's centre is and fully depends on the overall awareness or knowing of where that centre point is.

A little old lady takes small steps and falls over easily. This is not someone who has great awareness around their centre of mass and base of support. If she followed an AiM movement programme which allowed her to challenge her base of support, that awareness would change instantly and there would be a dramatic increase in her quality of life. This is not an uncommon story, nor is it a hypothetical example.

Postural and dynamic stability arises in a fully mobile environment. It arises only with a full experience of where one's centre is and fully depends on the overall awareness or knowing of where that centre point is

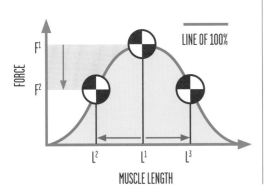

Stabilisation limits movement elsewhere in the body and changes our awareness of centre, dynamic equilibrium and balance

Challenging base of support

Optimal awareness in the muscle system comes when we challenge the perimeter of the base of support as opposed to happily sitting inside it. Another way of discussing this is to say "GET OUT OF YOUR COMFORT ZONE".

If you recognise your base of support and corresponding alignment of your centre of mass as your comfort zone – all that you currently know – then recognise also that this is the environment that your body will operate comfortably within on a daily basis.

Imagine that your centre of mass experienced every square inch of its base of support, and all the muscles and fascial lines associated with each position on the perimeter had the ability to control, stabilise and react to each position, whether to push you back into the comfort zone or allow you to venture off into a new and unexplored base of support shape.

Now imagine that your centre of mass only ever experienced dead centre of your base of support and wasn't allowed to stray from it – EVER. Minimal muscle movement – if any – pure neutral alignment, overall lack of awareness of movement, muscle and joint potential.

Can you see that this is the environment that is consistently taught as a base understanding in the world of fitness and therapy professionals to embrace and promote the concept of stabilisation?

Core stability in particular, but also knee, ankle, pelvis and shoulder stability. As I have suggested before, none of these movements can or should be

stabilised. Stabilisation limits movement elsewhere in the body and changes our awareness of centre, dynamic equilibrium and balance.

What could be worse than experiencing dead centre, however, is when people favour one side more than the other and have used stabilisation as an approach to protect any discomfort that arises from that dynamic posture. Stabilising the system without overriding the limp pattern does not make the situation better.

It's not unusual to see people favouring a stable pattern that is 'off-centre' and exemplified by a limp (you'd probably be surprised how many of you are actually limping around!).

I remember, once, offending a personal trainer at a talk I gave, by asking him if he had hurt himself as he limped towards the stage as a volunteer to stand on the foot scan. Ego suitably bruised, he had no idea of his natural gait and limp. Fortunately, the foot scan he volunteered for showed him and everyone else that, at least, I did have some idea of what I was talking about. It showed he was favouring one side and he was not even aware of it.

In this situation, when a person has a limp, the person's centre of mass spends more time in one specific area of the base of support. On a force plate we would see the centre of gravity resting in one of the four quadrants as opposed to in a central position during stance. We would also notice differences in the gait cycle of each foot since both feet function differently to each other. This naturally influences muscles and joints differently on one side of the body to the other. This is a pure definition of imbalance and is the most likely cause of your

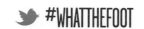

WHAT THE FOOT?

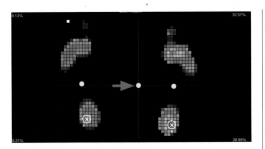

⬆ IMAGE TO SHOW CENTRE OF MASS FAVOURING ONE SIDE OF THE BODY

client's/patient's pain, discomfort and inhibition. Just what if we could stimulate the body to reorganise itself to bring the centre of mass back to centre and encourage each foot to work in the same way as each other?

It is not uncommon to see people whose muscle system is unwilling to receive a pelvis on the left-hand side and, consequently, the muscles on the right side are receiving it too much – the muscles on the right side become like a soggy trampoline that has lost its elasticity and can offer no return (a weak catapult effect). One side of the body is overworking and the other side of the body is underworking, creating asymmetric movement in the pelvis.

What if we taught that left side to receive the pelvis better? The person's pain could be in their knee, low back or shoulder and yet one major thing to deal with is this obvious movement-based flaw.

To teach the pelvis to travel around and experience all areas within and beyond the base of support in a pain-free environment would naturally re-educate the muscles around the pelvis to do their job better and instantly take the pressure off the affected inhibited joints or area of discomfort.

We use our three-dimensional approach to movement to challenge the brain's perception of its own base of support, and expand on what it currently conceives as its comfort zone by visiting, and going beyond, the perceived boundaries that have been put in place by the brain.

As discussed earlier, visiting the dark zone or unexplored areas of movement that exist due to inhibition and poor centre of mass alignment is one way of stimulating the brain to experience new ways of stance and movement. Once this is perceived as more useful, efficient and, crucially, pain free, it triggers the brain to access all ranges and utilise the new patterns that have been reinstalled, bringing balance to the system as a whole.

Stability vs mobility

Stability is one side of the coin; mobility is the other. Stability is a known concept for managing your pain. It resides on the one side of the proverbial coin. There is a biomechanical approach around postural sway (how the body moves in quiet standing) where sway can be viewed negatively, whereas I place enormous value on getting the body to enhance the sway so it may control that sway even better. I place value on the other side of the coin, which just so happens to be the side of mobility.

A note on the 'stability-mobility' spectrum here, representing opposite sides of the coin:

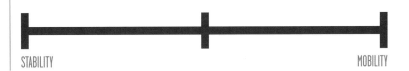

STABILITY   MOBILITY

WHAT THE FOOT?

By working at the mobility end of the spectrum you get BOTH – enhanced mobility AND enhanced stability

The stability end of the spectrum is based all around neutral and isolated approaches to minimise movement in specific structures in the body.

The mobility end of the spectrum is based on mobilising the centre of mass to challenge the base of support, encouraging skeletal motion to provide muscles with no option but to contract, and enabling joints to experience the movement potential they were blessed with.

By working at the stability end of the spectrum, you effectively limit movement in the system to create a strong and stable comfort zone for the body to function in.

By working at the mobility end of the spectrum, you promote movement in every joint, which stimulates reaction in the muscles and optimises the centre of mass over its base of support, effectively centring the body so it can access all ranges in all joints. Ironically, by working at the mobility end of the spectrum, you create stability in the system and therefore get BOTH – enhanced mobility AND enhanced stability with no TVA draw in sight.

In actual fact, the terms 'mobility' and 'stability' cannot be separated and is a classic example of the finding centre model.

Too much stability = reduced mobility
Too much mobility = reduced stability

Centre = where mobility naturally generates the stability in a balanced environment.

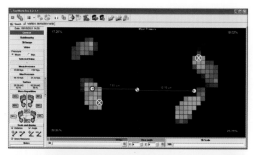

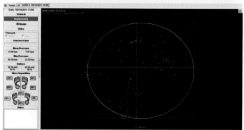

⬆ **STATIC SCAN OF 3 1/2-YEAR-OLD BOY ON A PERPETUAL WOBBLE (AS WE ALL ARE)**

The body has a natural way of being stable in a mobile environment. So, in fact, the body knows how to access the two sides of the coin perfectly. All babies, in fact, use this method as a way of learning how to walk. They wobble and wobble, activating the muscle system to gain an awareness of being upright. They challenge their base of support and explore their base of support until they can finally stand up, and then challenge it further until they can walk. They overcome the wobbliness and appear to become stable – whilst still wobbling around over their base of support.

Above is the static scan of my 3½–year–old boy and his stabilometry measurement; it looks like he's 'still learning to stand still', but he isn't, he's on a perpetual wobble – as we all are.

🐦 **#WHATTHEFOOT**

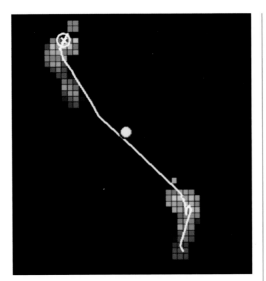

↑ DYNAMIC SCAN OF A 14-MONTH-OLD UTILISING HER GAIT RELATIVE BASE OF SUPPORT TO REMAIN UPRIGHT AND IN MOTION

And here above is a dynamic scan of my 14-month-old daughter just learning to walk. You can see evidence of the flow motion model that I discuss in Chapter 6 present in her gait (right foot) already at such a young age.

In terms of changing the focus from stability to mobility, I feel it important to add that the Pilates teachers who have taken the AiM courses love adding the movement concept into their programmes and experience large amounts of change in themselves as a result of the process – normally reported after one weekend. 3D Pilates? Of course. Bring it on!

Having said that, I can honestly say that of all the students on AiM courses and workshops so far, the worst bodies for movement practice and gait analysis are (eek!) Pilates teachers who have spent years training stability into their system, reducing movement in their pelvis and ribcage to have a super tight and stable core. The lack of movement in their bodies is visibly evident in their gait and foot scans and means that hip joints, shoulder joints and feet are over or underworking to compensate for the shortfall of mobility in the system as a whole.

Pilates gets its successes with pain by stabilising the system and limiting movement around the pain. This has naturally carried over into corrective exercise for personal trainers as well, and core stability has taken the whole world by storm!

My point is not that Pilates is bad or wrong, but that it forms part of a solution and we must embrace the two sides of the coin to get the best out of our clients. Some reformer classes and advanced Pilates certainly do go some way to developing that, which is fantastic.

CORE TRAINING

Right in the centre of the body lies the 'core'. The core has been described as the body minus the arms and legs, but most people – in particular the media and therefore your clients, too – still think of it as the area between the ribcage and the pelvis. To be stable in this area is everything!

I agree, yet the ideal approach for developing stability is through movement and not through stabilisation. Here's why:

SPINE

The spine is not a column, such as those in the image on the next page. It does, however, act as a column, taking into account the following definition:

WHAT THE FOOT?

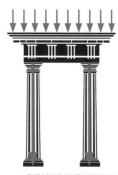

↑ THE SPINE ISN'T A COLUMN
AND THEREFORE SHOULD NOT
BE TREATED AS ONE

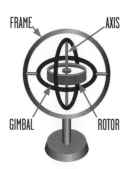

FRAME   AXIS

GIMBAL   ROTOR

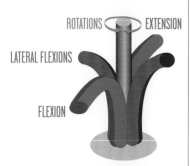

ROTATIONS   EXTENSION

LATERAL FLEXIONS

FLEXION

↑ THE SPINE HAS SIX MOTIONS
AVAILABLE TO IT AND SHOULD
BE TAUGHT TO ACCESS EACH

"A column or pillar in architecture and structural engineering is a vertical structural element that transmits, through compression, the weight of the structure above to other structural elements below." (Wikipedia)

I liken the spine to a gyroscope. Whilst it isn't a gyroscope per se, it is a three-dimensional structure that is designed to maintain overall orientation and balance of a system whilst acting as a column to disperse the weight of the ribcage, skull and shoulder girdle.

The image of the 'spinal gyroscope' (left) shows the three dimensionality of the spine. In the three dimensions we can see the spine flex and extend, laterally flex to the left and the right and rotate to the left and the right.

Each dimension has two opposing poles and a natural midpoint. The dimension of the sagittal plane, for example, incorporates flexion and extension, with the centre point being the optimal position at which the spine can equally access both ends of the spectrum.

We know full well that the spine should be able to both flex and extend and the optimal place from which to access both is the 'neutral' position or, as I call it, centre.

When we consider the remaining two dimensions, each one having two extremes either side of that 'neutral' centred position (left and right lateral flexions and rotations), it's plain to see that the spine is designed to move and not designed to be stabilised or locked into the neutral position. In order for the spine to fully experience its movement potential and

truly know its midpoint it has to be asked to move on a regular basis.

When the spine experiences this full three-dimensional potential, the following become a possibility:
- The more likely your spine is to access that centre point
- The greater freedom and awareness the muscles attached to your spine will have
- The more optimal the alignment of your spine will be

Walking around, it's plain to see that the general population favours the flexed spine. I can tell you that these people struggle to extend it, too. In fact, many people I work with (including fitness and therapy professionals) present with poor (if any) extension and uneven rotation through the spine in gait and often will favour rotation to one side over the other in isolated testing. The same goes for lateral flexion – favouring one side or limited in range on one or both sides.

If there is little or no rotation and one-sided or limited lateral flexion in one's spine, then the idea of stabilising that spine to minimise damage to it is extremely short-sighted. Would you really want to stabilise something that already doesn't move very well? Really? I hope you can see that if stability and mobility are on the same spectrum then a spine that lacks mobility ultimately needs mobilising, doesn't it?

Stabilising the core minimises the muscular experience of range and the muscular role in managing movement of the spine. What are muscles going to do if they don't have any

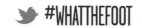

movement to decelerate? Nothing! Since if they have nothing to decelerate, there can't even be any activation as activation or concentric contraction would generate a movement that needs decelerating! Do you see the conundrum?

If all muscles attached onto the spine were to concentrically pull together, then theoretically the spine would not move – it would be stable and the effort involved in stabilising it in this way is exhausting. The body would soon adapt to find an easier way. This is how the body adapts and downgrades towards faulty postures – because they are easier to manage. Excessive focus on stabilisation, I'm sorry to say, can and does lead to this recurring situation.

Looking beyond the spinal gyroscope model to include the pelvis, the ribcage and shoulder girdle – all three-dimensional structures themselves – we begin to notice a vast array of muscles that all reach out from this 'core' and into the arms and legs. And as I said earlier, if it is to be true that when we move anything we move everything, then movement in the arms, legs and feet requires effective movement through the core structures as well; both structurally (bones) and functionally (muscles), too.

In motion, as the arms and legs swing and spiral, so must there be movement present in the spine, the core and the whole system.

In order to train the core for mobility, we simply have to create ways of mobilising the spinal gyroscope to demand the muscles to react in such a way that it kicks the core region into action. As I have said before, in this way we can give the muscles no option

but to contract and manage the spine, pelvis and ribcage as well as the legs and arms if we tailor the exercises in such a way.

If this sounds difficult, I urge you to take any 'core' exercise you can think of and ask the spine to travel through its three dimensions to access all ranges instead of keeping it still (please don't use any weights the first time) and compare the feeling and sensation with the stabilised exercise and you'll notice a huge difference. You can have a look at the section on the abdominals later in the book, where I guide you to work out the true role of that muscle. This will help you open your mind on mobilising your core.

I know what you are thinking:

"But what about injured clients who need stabilising?"

My simple answer is that we do not have a mechanism in the body that is set up to be stable: not the spine, not the core, not the diaphragm (imagine!), not the knee, not the ankle, not the scapula or the shoulder girdle!

Nothing.

If we try to keep our centre of mass still, we can't. If we try to minimise movement in a joint or set of joints (say the foot), we ask the body to move excessively elsewhere. The body will always overcompensate somewhere else for any movement inhibition.

Imagine I needed equal movement in each vertebrae for a healthy spine and the surgeon

In motion, as the arms and legs swing and spiral, so must there be movement present in the spine, the core and the whole system

WHAT THE FOOT?

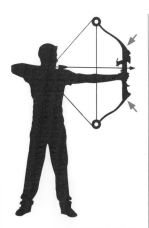

↑ THE STIFFENER PLATE ON THE BOW SIMPLY SHIFTS THE MOST MOBILE POINT ON THE BOW TO THE ENDS OF THE PLATE. A FUSED SPINE DOES THE SAME — INSTEAD OF ONE MOBILE JOINT (WHICH GETS FUSED), THERE ARE NOW TWO OTHER MOBILE JOINTS. SHOULD WE FUSE THEM AS WELL?

fused one of the vertebrae. What happens to the movement potential at that vertebrae — does it get fused as well? No, the next joints in the chain will begin to move even more to compensate for the lack of movement at the fusion.

Inhibiting movement at any point in the human body has this knock-on effect. If I can't move through my core I will overcompensate at the hip and shoulder joints. If I can't extend my thoracic spine, I will overcompensate in the cervical spine, lumbar spine and pelvis. If I can't supinate my feet I will compensate everywhere.

Everything orbits around centre: everything.

No planets fail to orbit the sun, hence my use of the word. Any movement in the body affects the position of the centre of mass and in order to maintain balance, the whole body moves and adapts itself around the centre of mass.

The centre of mass is constantly changing and so is the body. It's never, ever, ever still or stable.

If you do need to bring stability to a patient post-surgery or accident, it is essential to teach them mobility, too. At this point I'd like to remind you that to embrace both ends of the spectrum or both sides of the coin is the most effective way of working with the human body.

I often think that if movement is a way of challenging the comfort zone of a person to encourage advancement and growth, then stability could be used as a way of giving a comfort zone back to a post-operative patient/client. After all, you cannot challenge someone's comfort zone if they have no

awareness of one in the first place! You would then simply move from creating a comfort zone, to challenging it and expanding on it in their day-to-day environment.

In clients/patients who are not in this position, such as athletes in training or rehab, stabilisation, to me at least, is a crazy thing to waste your time doing with a player. In sports that involve movement — it's difficult to think of one that doesn't — our job as practitioners should be to challenge and develop the movement patterns that they use on the field of play, on the court or whatever environment they perform in. Even better than that, can you get close to doing it in the environment they perform in?

So many therapy departments that I have been in, or coaching faculties at professional clubs, are focused around this idea of stabilisation and localisation of single muscles or muscle groups without optimally reintegrating movement into the athletes (which for me is a huge WTF?) and challenging their awareness of required movement whilst connecting the dots so that the whole system can efficiently and effortlessly orbit around centre.

Ankle stability for a tennis player?
Hip stability for a footballer?
Core stability for a sprinter?
Shoulder stability for a cricketer?
Really?

Perhaps this is why we see so many sub-patellar straps on tennis players or hamstring injuries in footballers. All I know is that, in my experience, giving access to movement for these players has a significant reduction in future injury and a quicker return to the playing field. Theoretically, priceless...

 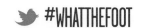

Finding centre

Finding centre is essentially how you can teach the body to heal itself. There is no requirement to guide someone into movement in a controlled manner with a 'do this, do that' approach. I understand that this is deemed safe and considerate, but it does not help your clients break through to a new level of wellbeing. It does not stimulate the brain – more, it becomes a way of managing people's problems and keeping pain at bay when, as it happens, there is a very real and distinct possibility of blowing their pain out of the water. But you, as a therapist, cannot do that – you, as a therapist, have to let go of that very ideal. Of all the tricks you have ever learnt, the most important one may be to know that you can purely facilitate the healing in someone and the healing has to take place in the person who owns the pain.

Introducing movement and understanding centre of mass and how the structures orbit around it creates an environment for the brain and nervous system to reorganise what it currently perceives as normal to a higher new state of normal where things don't hurt anymore. You, as a therapist, can not know where that is for everybody – you can't. You can have a hunch, but you will always be stabbing in the dark somewhat. The truth is that the only person capable of accessing the healing, the state of balance and symmetry that potentially eliminates the pain, is the person themself. So rather than teach centre (i.e. neutral spine), I teach you to find centre by mobilising the whole structure to reveal what is possible, opening new pathways, awakening dormant muscles and revealing new structural motion to a body that has simply got into bad habits.

IN SUMMARY

▶ **The relationship the body has with centre is integral to its functional capabilities.**

▶ **The centre of mass and base of support play a huge role in defining postural and dynamic potential.**

▶ **Balance is really mass management or how you manage your centre of mass.**

▶ **Balance in terms of alignment is an appreciation of end ranges of motion in all dimensions of motion available to the body.**

▶ **Balance is not wobbling around on one leg. Balance being the opposite of imbalance requires equilibrium to be present in a dynamic environment.**

▶ **To overlook one's centre is to overlook the usage of that person's body in all activities they carry out.**

▶ **A perfect example for big rule #3 is not to accept that standing on one leg is a challenge for the individual. Shift your mindset to one that is prepared to challenge the way that person stands on one leg.**

▶ **When all centres come into alignment, balance becomes easy.**

Finding centre is essentially how you can teach the body to heal itself. There is no requirement to guide someone into movement in a controlled manner with a 'do this, do that' approach. I understand that this is deemed safe and considerate, but it does not help your clients break through to a new level of wellbeing

WHAT THE FOOT?

AiM does
not only
deal with the
biomechanics
or what
muscle
does what,
it delves
deeper into
the inner
function of
the human

CASE STUDY

I was introduced to AiM through ailments of my own. I had met Gary at a sports convention and had an interesting conversation. Not knowing each other's background, simply as this was our first encounter, it was evident to me the synergy in our core messages. Weirdly, we were from two different aspects of the industry, or so I thought at the time.

I am a professional tennis coach and it was 'competition' season for me personally with the National Club League event in full swing. I was playing some tough matches and having some serious issues post-match with my left leg. Hip flexor was incredibly painful with the pain radiating down my left side, resulting in some startling swelling in my left ankle. In a sheep-like manner I followed the route that others would: bit of ice, see a massage therapist and simply complain! It then came about, maybe fate, maybe I was getting smarter, but I called AiM. I knew deep down I should meet with Mr Ward anyway and we had discussed a 'show and tell' possibility. We met, and I am one happy bunny!

I spent a whole 10 minutes working with Mr Ward and the ever common feeling of walking on air is the most prevalent memory of the treatment. However, being a cynic, or as others might say 'a royal pain in the ass', the proof would be in the pudding. I had a big match against a player ranked inside the top 1,000 in the world and I knew it would be tough. Three sets and a couple of hours later I was sat grinning like a Cheshire cat. Not only due to the victory, but also because this dreadful onset of pain and swelling was missing.

Where was it? The next day provided the answer as I woke up with sore hamstrings and glutes. Extensor chain! Had I finally started to use the relevant muscle groups? I had to find out more about this and so enter level 1.

Subsequently, I have completed all of the AiM courses and it has been a revelation in my thinking and approach to the development of tennis players. I have been able to form a philosophy of coaching with a deep understanding of the functionality of the body and the requirements in producing tennis strokes. I can analyse these strokes to create movement exercises to promote technical learning and integrate this into a tactical learning environment in order to allow my students the ability to explore the full potential of their possible game.

AiM does not only deal with the biomechanics or what muscle does what, it delves deeper into the inner function of the human. It taps into the self and delivers it from evil, guiding it down a route of enlightenment both mentally and physically. AiM never judges a body, but takes it by the hand and enhances the experience in pain-free, three-dimensional space. Feelings of joy, freedom and possibility result from learning and using AiM, and it has taken my humble teaching of tennis to new levels. It should be that every sports coach has experienced AiM and many will then realise that their coaching has been missing something.

Mike Crooks, Tennis and Sports Coach, creator of HotSpot
www.thetennisengineer.wordpress.com

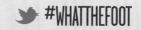

BIG RULE #4: PERCEIVED CENTRE DICTATES MOVEMENT, POSTURE, PAIN AND POTENTIAL

Student Clare informed me of the problems she had and limitations that existed in her body, so that I would be aware of her limitations on the course the following weekend.

She had one leg longer than the other and had been managing it for a long time. Consider the impact a leg length discrepancy can have on your centre, the adaptations in your joint alignment and the subsequent balance in the muscle and fascial system. This is something we have to deal with in life and the brain has an incredible power to make your body feel 'normal' despite the obvious inhibition.

Clare's leg was clearly longer on one side. She had adapted her whole body to accommodate this. It affected the way she walked and the way she played golf... and not in a good way I might add. As a demonstration of the power of the work, I borrowed her for a pelvic and leg length assessment. Scan it... Identify it... Solve it... One or two movements later and her leg length difference had been corrected. Not just for 10 minutes, but for as long as I have known her. These movements changed her perception of what is 'normal' in her body.

I remember describing to Clare how her story of one leg being longer than the other had always been just that – a story. Mere perception; and in actual fact was not true at all. A big hearty thanks to all the conventional therapists who failed to dig deeper to find the route of the problem, was her first response.

Clare is today an exceptional AiM graduate as she now recognises the power of how our perception of what is normal affects us physically and emotionally on a day-to-day basis.

Perception

Perception is an interesting word. You currently perceive that everything you do in this world is 'right' – otherwise you wouldn't do it. Behind everything you do also lies a positive intention.

What you perceive as normal for yourself, somebody else has the capacity to judge and decide that, to them at least, it is abnormal. Someone else could conceive what you perceive to be the right thing to say as a very bad thing indeed. Awkward...

Your perceptions form the way you are and encompass what feels normal or right for you in the world. If you had a bad experience as a child around spiders, you may have subconsciously set up a system to protect you from them – a system grounded in the desire for survival (your positive intention), which may come in the form of a phobia. I don't fear spiders, but you might. I definitely think that's odd, but for you it could be completely normal.

It's the same in the body. You are the way you are. Your body presents itself daily in the most efficient way it can – even where pain is present. Your pain is present as a result of current movement inhibitions or previous compensations in the system as a whole. An extrinsic accident (something that happened through no fault of your own body – like being hit by an external obstacle, for example) can also lead to a protective response in the subconscious system.

What you perceive as normal for yourself, somebody else has the capacity to judge and decide that, to them at least, it is abnormal. Someone else could conceive what you perceive to be the right thing to say as a very bad thing indeed. Awkward...

WHAT THE FOOT?

Our dysfunction is actually pure functionality

The way you present yourself, the way you walk and move, feels entirely normal for you, but could appear to someone else as dysfunctional – i.e. your physical therapist. Left alone for long enough, even a limp or inability to twist to the right will begin to feel normal.

I hate that word by the way: 'dysfunction'.

FUNCTION VS DYSFUNCTION

Dysfunction is often used to describe a joint that doesn't have full range or a muscle that doesn't activate when it should. Ordinarily it describes something that doesn't work properly!

Yet this is a global system we are talking about – a system that, no matter what life throws at it, simply knows how to function perfectly all the time. Your body will do whatever it takes to optimise its movement patterns and posture regardless of the environment it operates in.

Your body and the bodies of your clients are 100% functional all of the time. So let's imagine that you have a so-called dysfunctional hip. Is it biomechanically incapable of doing what it could? Or is it just underperforming as a global consequence of everything else that is happening in the body?

We have already said that if one joint underperforms then all others have to compensate to maintain balance in the system. This compensation is actually pure functionality, yet it creates a perception to the trained eye of 'dysfunction'.

Dysfunction is earmarked by the body's ability to self-correct within the skeletal framework to maintain balance in the system. The problem is that the self-correction is a correction away from normal,

often in compensation or adaptation – altering posture, for example, to maximise performance.

Dysfunction is actually something we can be grateful for as it assists us in overcoming our imbalances and creating a new functional space for us to operate in.

Dysfunction arises out of a need to look at the body in isolation, under the laser. We know that a joint should operate in a certain way, and when it doesn't we judge it and give it the big 'D' label.

Looking at the body globally, under the light bulb, we can see the whole picture and come to an understanding of why that hip may operate in such a way. In actual fact, the body is choosing that hip to operate in the 'dysfunctional' way to fully facilitate the continuation and accessibility of function.

If you take adaptation to mean a whole body change in how it operates to keep functioning optimally then dysfunction could be described as an adaptation from one functional space to another. On the bell curves highlighted on pages 76 and 77, we always sit on the curve, the line of 100%. Even though we remain functional and are able to go about our daily tasks, our force output or potential is reduced – so we can still do it, but just not as efficiently as is physically possible, given the parameters available in the human body. Always functional, never dysfunctional.

Likewise, a dysfunctional muscle is simply reacting negatively to a downturn in performance of the whole skeleton (big rule #2).

If you judge the body to be in a dysfunctional state, as many conventional practitioners do (I'm sure it's

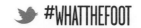

just a language thing), then it is my humble opinion that you have failed to respect the awesome power of the human body and its ability to adapt to anything and everything that we throw at it.

Its ability to respond to changes to the external environment and within its internal environment in order to keep you moving is nothing short of phenomenal. The body does this every second of every day in all situations. It responds to changes in environment, ground, speed, competition, habit and pain among other things.

Injury or inhibition demands this very response from the subconscious brain: the body requires the brain to discover the most efficient pathway of movement and posture for the current state of the body... and quickly!

It always follows the path of least resistance. The path of least resistance is the most efficient, most energy conserving and most effortless environment it can operate in when taking all factors (external and internal) into account.

Your body is working optimally ALL of the time. It is perfect. It responds to changes by balancing the joint system through a tension–based exchange in the fascial system, conserving energy wherever and whenever possible.

If the body is working 100% all of the time, then fitness and therapy professionals are going to have a difficult time changing it. For example, you cannot ask the body to function at 110%, and there's no way you'd entertain asking it to work at anything less. So our role as practitioners is not to CHANGE the body, but to CHALLENGE it to recognise new ways

of functioning, with the aim, ultimately, of pressing the big reset button to return the body back towards optimal performance.

The only possibility that arises through the medium of challenge, therefore, is to transform the way it works within the 100%. Reorganising the way it operates within the 100% framework is only achievable by bringing both sides of the coin together.

Einstein says that "Energy can neither be created nor destroyed, it can only be transformed". In other words, we cannot add anything or take anything away from the human body, we can only transform the way it operates within the 100%.

The human body is functioning perfectly 100% of the time – remember that if nothing else!

If you are limping, it could be said that your limp is the effortless way in which your body goes about its business (or, more accurately, it's how the body sets itself up so you can go about your business).

Homeostasis or balance is achieved effortlessly in the world around us. The transformation from summer to autumn is effortless. In order to operate by design the world must operate in a state of balance. Even when it appears not to be in balance, it actually is, all of the time.

One way of approaching this is to ask: "How does the apparently dysfunctional part of the system serve the system as a whole?" The answer can only be a positive one – one that brings balance and harmony to a system in free fall.

> *"Energy can neither be created nor destroyed, it can only be transformed."*
> **Albert Einstein**

WHAT THE FOOT?

Dynamic equilibrium is a perpetual state of balance that ebbs and flows from one side of the see-saw to the other. Never still, always in motion. Always orbiting around centre

DYNAMIC EQUILIBRIUM

Dynamic equilibrium is a perpetual state of balance that ebbs and flows from one side of the see-saw to the other. Never still, always in motion. Always orbiting around centre. When we take snapshots of any situation we see the situation as it is in that moment. When we pull back and look at the bigger picture we see it for what it is – we see which way the momentum is flowing and where it has been, why things have changed and the harmony it brings to the situation.

For the body, it is the same. The dynamic equilibrium is evident when the centre of mass orbits around a static base, facilitating balance and yet is never static.

Hair analysis assessments used to frustrate the hell out of me. It would tell me that calcium is high relative to potassium and that means 'x', but since it was taken from one sample, there could be no evidence of what was really going on. Could it be that the calcium was moving further away from the potassium at the time of the snapshot or could it have been moving closer? The truth of which would completely change the outcome of the test. The perpetual state of hormones and chemicals in the body is one of motion – never static and always designed to bring balance to a global system. In this situation, simply adding potassium to the scene would change nothing: what's the bigger picture? What do you have to do to that body to bring it back into balance, where stress is simply less?

Dynamic equilibrium is a point that is moving (dynamic) around an optimum central balance point (equilibrium).

Is it possible to be purely centred? The possibility, if it arises at all, can only be possible for a very fleeting moment. The key then is to ensure that movement around this point of balance is minimal, but present. The further we stray from this point, the greater the tension in the system (physical or hormonal) will be and the greater the problems that can arise.

PERCEIVED CENTRE

Back to movement then; it could be described that true centre is our point of maximum efficiency where all planes, ranges and directions of movement are available. Thus it becomes easier and effortless to make any movement a reality.

If my centre of mass sits over my left foot there is a greater amount of effort required to bring my centre of mass over my right foot, as it now has further to travel in space than when I am in centre. This stance is accompanied by an orbital reaction of the skeleton to this stance, i.e. the skeleton wholly adjusts its posture to maintain balance with all the weight now sitting so far to the left. The result will be that the skeleton experiences a whole shift of itself to facilitate this new position of the centre of mass (shift your weight from left to right to feel yourself orbiting around your centre).

In this case, a practitioner will normally recognise dysfunction, altered posture, coupled with a selection of joints with inhibited range, as well as a bunch of inactive and overactive muscles. Whilst it makes sense in book form to suggest that all we have to do is get all of the joints to move as they are supposed to and have the muscles react normally in response, it is sadly not viewed that way in the conventional practices of rehabilitation or therapy. What I mean by this is it is more likely that this particular client would be treated on several localised levels as opposed to one global level. The former would ultimately

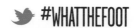

not target the alignment of the centre of mass or even believe that to impact upon this is actually possible. So traditionally, we stabilise and get strong in this posture.

Where the practitioner sees dysfunction, I see pure functionality, and choose to respect that this is the position that the body itself has chosen to optimise efficient function in its current environment.

I also know a 'perceived centre' when I see one – a habitual state taken on by the brain to record this posture as necessary for survival.

Perceived centre describes the posture that feels normal to you and the physical self-awareness that you have around this posture. I'll be blunt: it feels normal to you, but looks abnormal to someone else – normally a bodywork practitioner! We see everything – the slightest glitch in alignment or anomaly in posture.

When your perception of centre is, in actual fact, centre itself, then your movement, your posture and your potential are maximised and your pain and inhibitions are minimised.

In most cases, what actually feels normal to modern man is the altered posture he chooses to stand in, which the brain has predetermined to allow for maximum movement potential. In this state, your maximum movement potential is naturally limited, compared to your optimum movement potential, and yet it represents what is maximally available to you now, given the altered posture on display.

For example, most people have over-pronated feet. They just get on with it. When was the last time you woke up grumpy and said "Oh, if only my feet weren't so over-pronated!"?

The thing about over-pronated feet is that they simply cannot allow the body to perform optimally as it appears to have been designed, thus it must settle for generating maximum functionality possible, given the parameters it has to deal with today.

So it responds in a variety of ways – all of which are possible:
- Feet turned out
- Knees hyper-extended
- Pelvis tilted forwards or backwards
- Spinal kyphosis
- Deactivated glutes
- Forward head posture
- Slumped ribcage/protracted shoulder girdle

If you didn't notice by the way, I just described the masses. These people walk into your gym and clinic every day. It could even be you!

When the feet are introduced to a larger amount of movement than they are ordinarily used to, we notice the following:
- Joint alignment of the foot improves
- The muscles have more range and react quicker
- Posture as a whole benefits enormously

On the down side, if one foot is flatter than the other the body responds in the frontal plane by shifting the centre of mass laterally, driving the pelvis sideways, causing a side bend in the spine, carrying a functional scoliosis in the spine, overtightening a groin, tightness in one side of the neck and/or a variety of unnecessary rotations in the system (rotated ribcage, rotated pelvis, oppositely rotated hips, etc). Nightmare!

> *Where the practitioner sees dysfunction, I see pure functionality, and choose to respect that this is the position that the body itself has chosen to optimise efficient function in its current environment*

WHAT THE FOOT?

TRANSVERSE PLANE ADAPTATION

FRONTAL PLANE ADAPTATION

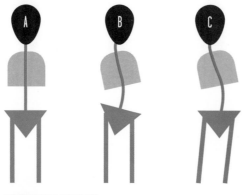

SAGITTAL PLANE ADAPTATION

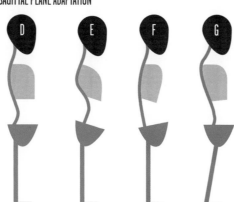

A FRONTAL PLANE NEUTRAL
B HIP HIKED ON LEFT
C HIP SHIFTED TO RIGHT
D SAGITTAL PLANE NEUTRAL
E ANTERIOR TILT OF PELVIS
F POSTERIOR TILT OF PELVIS
G ANTERIOR SHIFT OF PELVIS
H TRANSVERSE PLANE NEUTRAL
I PELVIS ROTATED RIGHT,
RIBCAGE LEFT
J PELVIS ROTATED LEFT,
RIBCAGE RIGHT
K BOTH RIBCAGE AND PELVIS
ROTATED IN SAME DIRECTION
(IN OPPOSITION TO THE FEET)

If all that can come from just having pronated feet (and one more so than the other), imagine what could happen if you had any of the other hundreds of pathologies or inhibitions charted through history in your body.

Actually, and thankfully, not a huge amount more, I can tell you. I regularly draw up all available possibilities of 'dysfunctional' postures on a side of A3 paper for all groups I teach to see. There are only a handful in which all pathologies would exist and

therefore only a handful of ways the body can react when it is upright on two feet with a primary goal of keeping the centre of mass inside the base of support, as illustrated to the left.

Finally some simplicity! Or not?

If you are thinking that the number of adaptations the body can make when upright and in motion are so minimal, then perhaps that minimises the number of options I have to get it back to ideal centre?

Then you would be right.

Perceived centre is a reaction to change in the body that creates a reaction in the skeleton and has a downgrade in performance attached to it whilst increasing the potential for pain and risk of injury.

On a very base level, my goal is to change your own perception of your own centre.

Let's have a quick look at that diagrammatically.

Diagram A represents the distribution of physical potential and the corresponding opportunity that creates. As your physical performance is minimised through altered posture, the opportunity you experience is equally minimised.

Diagram B balances the two sides of the coin and brings the centre to life. In centre we have maximum opportunity in the human body and the closer we are to physical centre, the higher our physical potential is. To be closer to centre and experience our higher potential, we must move towards and orbit around a state of dynamic equilibrium or balance.

WHAT THE FOOT?

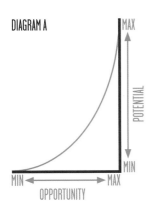

DIAGRAM A

POTENTIAL

MAX

MIN

MIN ← → MAX
OPPORTUNITY

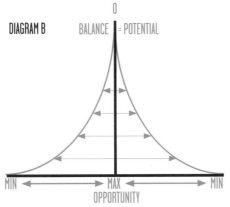

DIAGRAM B

0
BALANCE = POTENTIAL

MIN ← → MAX   MAX ← → MIN
OPPORTUNITY

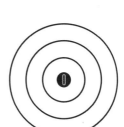

DIAGRAM C

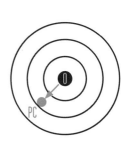

DIAGRAM D

PC

The further we move away from centre, the lower our physical potential becomes, and our physical opportunity naturally reduces along with it. We could look at this in a number of ways, basically summarised by the following:

- An increase in potential is synonymous with an increase in performance, a reduction in effort and an effortless life.
- A decrease in potential is accompanied by increased risk of injury, higher possibilities of pain and a guaranteed reduction in performance or output.

As our physical potential peaks, our opportunities within our body increase, too.

I cannot physically leap outside of this curve, but will simply operate along it. I call it the line of 100%, or the line of function.

Diagram B shows you a more realistic look at this chart when we consider both sides of centre, and can be expanded on further when we look at the full three dimensionality of the system.

The performance peak in diagram B, or should I say where peak performance is available for all, is at

point O. When looked down upon from above, this chart looks like concentric circles with this point O appearing at perfect centre (diagram C).

The dot in the middle represents true centre and any journey towards the outer rings is a movement away from centre, and a reduction in opportunity occurs. We should note here that in a state of dynamic equilibrium, our centre would be oscillating around the ideal centre point in order to generate stability in the system, as described in big rule #3. Perceived centre is when the actual centre point around which we oscillate is no longer in the centre point, but has moved away, without us noticing. This can be seen represented by the blue dot in diagram D.

Back to our potential/opportunity chart, we now see this blue dot as a new point representing perceived centre — and we shift to a new centre line on the chart, which makes for new opportunity and new potential. Sadly, it's not good news!

The scenario we see here (as shown on page 94) is basically a 'leap' from one physical state to another — from centre to a perception of centre. This often goes unnoticed and the brain accommodates for

The dot in the middle represents true centre and any journey towards the outer rings is a movement away from centre, and a reduction in opportunity occurs

WHAT THE FOOT?

DIAGRAM E

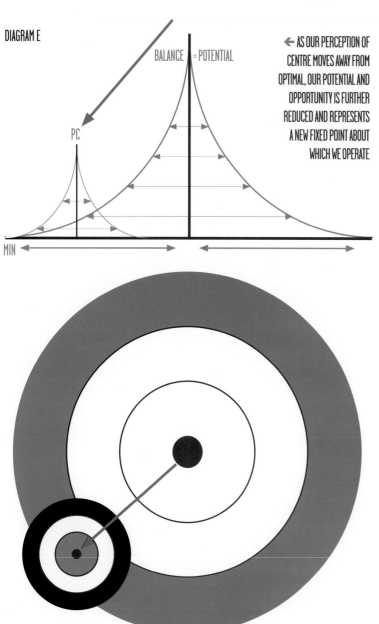

BALANCE = POTENTIAL

PC

MIN

← AS OUR PERCEPTION OF
CENTRE MOVES AWAY FROM
OPTIMAL, OUR POTENTIAL AND
OPPORTUNITY IS FURTHER
REDUCED AND REPRESENTS
A NEW FIXED POINT ABOUT
WHICH WE OPERATE

it instantly in the name of function. Here at point PC, the brain has a perception of optimal balance, despite the accompanying reduction in opportunity and potential. Again, looking down on this diagram from above, we can see the leap demonstrated in the circles below it in diagram E.

The blue dot migrates from centre and becomes fixed. As it wanders farther into the blue area, the effort to manage the system and keep it functional in its normal way becomes too great, so the system changes; downgrades its software to make for an effortless life. It leaps to the circle next to it, the new perceived centre: notice the circle is smaller to match the size of the base of the triangle in the top half of the diagram.

If the person is unlucky enough to journey from blue through grey and into black in the second circle, we might see further leaps into yet new physical states: each one affording us less and less mobility, potential and opportunity whilst facilitating the possibility of greater discomfort.

These changes take milliseconds. You wouldn't even notice them unless the cause of the leap was an accident, for example, which leaped you straight into the second circle. The question then is does your recovery and rehabilitation get you back to the centre in the first circle, enabling you to access peak performance, or keep you in the second circle, managing the problem and keeping pain at bay, in the land of compensation where it is a constant battle to recover your fitness?

Reverse compensation
Ultimately, it is your perception and awareness around your centre of mass and how you manage

that, and thus the whole skeleton, that dictates your physical wellbeing. It's just a brain thing, a mind thing – and you all know that it's possible to change your minds, don't you? As hard as it first might appear, I believe that change happens in an instant, and if we can go from normal to limping in a fraction of a second, I believe we can go from limping to normal, just as quickly. No six-week process – just a biomechanical quantum leap to a new and better you: a leap back through the circles to peak performance.

This backwards leap through the circles is overriding patterns of movement that were laid down to compensate for inhibited movement in the body. It takes no time at all to compensate for pain, like I just said; it's a fraction of a second, no more. What if we can reverse that compensation? What if the brain doesn't need six to eight weeks to work its way back to 'normal'? The speed of reaction to movement is akin to reversing these compensations. Milliseconds, not months.

You may have heard of peeling the layers of an onion back to get to the core; it's the same here, each circle representing another layer of the onion. Using movement and an application of the five big rules, we are able to challenge the body to find new centres, thus leaving an old centre behind, peeling back a layer of the onion whilst experiencing new freedom in the body.

What's important is that each layer or new circle represents a new perception of your own body. Your body feels different, you know something has happened, changed even, but you're not quite sure what. The brain is challenged by the sudden shift, it makes you smile. How can such a simple movement evoke such feelings and emotion? Your body ultimately knows where that centre point is – the one you've been avoiding ever since falling out of the tree as a child – and it longs to find it again, knowing at that point there is a chance of being out of pain and a chance of accessing higher performance states. Clients always report the same things: they feel lighter, they feel like they are using their whole foot, they feel floaty, they feel like they are taking in more oxygen, finding it easier to breathe, they feel taller, grounded, balanced and (everyone's favourite) centred! In essence, their compensations have been reversed.

What I have presented above is purely conceptual and normally assists in the understanding of the process we take clients through during a movement session. It's an awareness of how far away from centre the client is. To notice that people have poor posture – yet remain unaware of it – really highlights that, in actual fact, we are in a perceptual state of balance where things 'feel' normal, yet to the trained eye, these bodies are clearly not doing the job they could be doing.

I see our job as therapists to reset the systems that are responsible for the body to return to a state of 'real' normal, where the body is working as designed and no longer in a compensatory way at all.

Seeing as change does happen instantly as opposed to over a period of time, I have searched for the ways to encourage the brain to take these quantum leaps from one underperforming state to a higher performing state in as short a time frame as possible and the upshot has always been that when I do this, pain and problems simply drop away. Total body transformations are genuinely possible.

No six-week process – just a biomechanical quantum leap to a new and better you

"The effect of each level is to organise and control the information on the level below it. Changing something on an upper level changes things on the lower levels; changing something on a lower level could but would not necessarily affect the upper levels." (Dilts.)

When your clients present themselves in one of the postures outlined on page 92, or even a combination of two or more of them, they are presenting themselves as off-centre, with a need to peel back layers and layers of life's physical adaptations. Each posture represents a static or dynamic pattern that is missing from their daily movement and stance.

If the brain was to know the value and benefit of using these missing patterns that can create higher levels of efficiency and performance, it would use them wouldn't it? Of course it would. So why aren't we simply reintroducing tried-and-tested movement patterns to our clients' bodies for the brains to perceive a whole new centre and new way of functioning?

Once again, I personally think the answer lies in our interest to point the laser and find out what is going on in the lower levels. Remember the logical levels quote? We need to work on the higher levels to impact the lower, which is where we are so keen to look:

"The effect of each level is to organise and control the information on the level below it. Changing something on an upper level changes things on the lower levels; changing something on a lower level could but would not necessarily affect the upper levels." (Dilts.)

Back to Clare, who had a real leg length discrepancy, or so she thought – in actual fact, all she had suffered from in reality was insufficient insight into her problem; she had accepted it and henceforth remained in this perceived state of balance.

I set myself a simple challenge of testing her body (and brain) to see if she really did have a leg

length discrepancy or if it was simply her perception of centre.

I tested her brain through her own body, acknowledging that the two entities are one and the same, as inseparable as the foot and the pelvis.

On day two, we checked the pelvis for alignment anomalies and asked Clare to volunteer. We checked the height of both PSIS (posterior superior iliac spine) points on the pelvis and she clearly displayed that one was significantly higher than the other and also one knee was bent and the other locked straight – all indicators that she could have one leg longer than the other.

In simple AiM fashion, the PSIS that was dropped needed to be raised so as to be level and balanced. So I created an exercise, based on gait, incorporating all the joints in the kinetic chain, that would cause exactly that response if indeed her legs were really the same length.

Thirty seconds later the whole group could see that her pelvis was aligned – something it had not been for many years. Clare obviously could not believe it and the immediate reaction was 'why hasn't anyone else done that before?'

The simple answer is because most everyone is still looking at the isolated and static-based environment that we think tells the story of anatomy. You only have to bump into the 'functional trainers' and the yogis of this world to see an interest in integrated and global anatomy. Yet the philosophy and simplicity of AiM is what makes the difference in many of these scenarios.

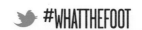

WHAT THE FOOT?

Most functional trainers, corrective exercise specialists and professional therapists are not aware that the body has a self-corrective mechanism of its own. Most of them probably believe that they, themselves, are the likely cause of their clients' successes. Yet those of you in the personal coaching industry or NLP (neurolinguistic programming) world will recognise that change occurs from within and no matter what you throw at the body or the mind, it will only change if it suits that person's body (and/or mind). If all parameters that led to the downgrade in function are eliminated, the body will naturally shift to a higher plane, balancing performance and opportunity with efficiency.

Following these five big rules we get the body to do its own healing. No egos. No dramas. If the body wants to change and you put the right parameters in place, locate the causative factors and integrate the whole system using a methodology of movement (something your body likes to do very much), it's just like hitting the reset button on the system and starting again.

I asked Clare if she had ever considered that her leg length difference was simply a 'story' in her own mind? She had not. I asked her if she was willing to let go of the notion that one leg was longer than the other and she had no choice — it was clear for all to see. She was in balance.

Is she grateful that we managed to hit the reset button on her body? You bet she is!

Symmetry and pain?
I'd like to acknowledge here the many people who have questioned this idea that symmetry holds hands with a pain-free system. I personally believe that pain cannot be present in a truly balanced system. And yet pain need not be present in an imbalanced system either — there are other factors at play that bring pain to the fore. What I would say is that the more asymmetrical we are, the greater the chance of there being some pain in the system. Either way, in a balanced or unbalanced state, it's important for us to recognise that the body has adopted a perception of its own centre, a perception of its most optimal posture and movement capabilities, and sets this in stone. It is this perception, for example, that hides away the fact that we are limping from our conscious brain. A limp is simply representative of an imbalance, which left alone and stabilised would create a limp forever more.

That limp will reach up into the body, demanding compensations throughout that could lead to pain. A simple approach to assess and challenge the joints in the limping leg would lead to a change in the brain's understanding of how to use the leg (and the whole body) differently, which naturally opens the body up to new possibilities for movement and daily life. This is a change in our brain's perception of what the body can do; if it hurts less or lends itself to freer movement and a slide up the bell curve to peak performance, then it's highly likely the brain will hang on to the new patterns of movement. Noticeably, symmetry will always be enhanced and pain reduced, if not eliminated.

If the body wants to change and you put the right parameters in place, it's just like hitting the reset button on the system and starting again

WHAT THE FOOT?

IN SUMMARY

- Dysfunction is pure functionality.
- Our perception of what is optimal dictates the posture we carry and movement patterns we access.
- Movement patterns aren't faulty – they are the patterns we choose to give us access to daily activities.
- Perception of centre is a person's awareness of the most efficient way of operating on a day-to-day basis, given the functional and skeletal parameters in place.
- Compensation is our brain's way of adapting to a new perception of centre that has been triggered by change in the physical system due to external or internal challenges.
- A shift in our perception of centre increases or decreases opportunity available to us in this body, exposes us to a risk of pain or, conversely, the possibility of high performance.
- Tragically, conventional approaches aim to support and bolster the downgrade rather than be open to a whole new shift back to more optimal states.
- Centre is centre: it's what the brain adds value to. To optimise it requires a challenge to the whole system.

BIG RULE #5: PERFECTION IS HARDWIRED AND COMES PRE-INSTALLED

This chapter gets a little more complex and I hope I have made it as accessible as possible in writing. It might help you to read it slowly, be patient as you reread various paragraphs, and I suggest you feel free to return back to it time and again to see if it reads differently as you absorb more of the material that is still to come in the book. The shift from body to brain is a critical leap in your engagement of the movement-based approach. The fact that your body is hardwired to a) self-optimise at any given moment and b) know where its true centre or balance point is, is kind of understood by professionals, but I would suggest not fully taken on. This also adds to this chapter in a way that may make rereading it again and again highly recommended.

In the four case studies that precede each of the four big rules above, I'd like to make clear that the change that occurred in their body was not a short-term fix, but was actually a long-term transformation of the way their body works: a complete rewiring of the brain, nervous system and musculoskeletal system. Put another way, a complete alteration in the perception of their own bodies.

This can only occur if the brain has an innate or inbuilt interpretation of what this rewiring would look like. In essence, these clients were not introduced to new movement patterns, rather more they were simply reintroduced to old movement patterns that were more effective.

The change and transformation that is consistently referred to in this book is only possible when we

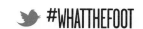

cease to think in the conventional and traditional way. Each case study subject had their whole body begin to operate in a completely different state to the one where the pain and limitations were present. It is in this state that things began to change for each client.

A bonus accompaniment for each is the mental shift that was experienced as a result of the work. As the tension relationships shift in the body, so they shift in the brain, too, creating a completely new space in which higher states of performance are instantly made available.

Perfect balance
Where conventional therapy potentially lets itself down is where it fails to get the body and brain to completely use the whole physical system in a different way.

If the body functions 100% all of the time, can we agree that if there are no inhibitions in the body, then that 100% is the ultimate optimal state for the body to be in?

In a downgrade of the physical system – a new perceived centre perhaps – the body works hard to maintain normal function. Sometimes overworking in certain areas and underperforming in others.

This equates to both joints and muscles. If one joint is restricted in its movement, another will have to allow more movement to bring balance to the system.

In the same way, if you have a fused spine, the joints at the end of the fusion must access the mobility lost in the fused vertebrae, rendering these vertebrae at risk. Cheers, Doc!

Equally, if you are hypermobile somewhere in the body it's most likely you are hypomobile in other areas of the body – all in the name of perfect balance.

Muscles, too, follow this thought process: skeletal alignment and movement potential dictates muscle length. When there is muscle shortening in the body, it stands to reason that there must be muscle lengthening somewhere, too. This is where the reciprocal inhibition concept arose.

Yet there are many occasions, again when assessed upright and in motion, that this rule breaks down, and there are moments where we see, for example, quads and hamstrings all lengthening at once to decelerate a specific movement elsewhere in the body – say, pronation in the suspension phase of gait when the foot is placed flat on the ground and pronating.

What is also possible, when looking at three dimensions of movement potential within a single muscle, is that muscles themselves can both lengthen and shorten in different dimensions.

So the following becomes possible:
- to shorten muscle fibres in all three planes of movement
- to shorten muscle fibres in two planes and lengthen in one
- to shorten muscle fibres in one plane and lengthen in two
- or lengthen in all three planes!

Such is the complexity and unpredictable nature of the human body.

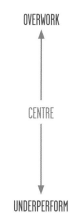

OVERWORK

CENTRE

UNDERPERFORM

WHAT THE FOOT?

A reiteration of all that has been said before is that muscles will simply align themselves with the position of the centre of mass in both static and dynamic environments, and if this means lengthening in some dimensions and shortening in others to do so, then so be it! Who are we to judge or predict what the body needs to do to optimise functionality and maintain integrity in its own wholesome system?

We can, however, look at it with our eyes and mind wide open to discover what we need to do, in order to balance the system and bring balance to the tension in the muscles.

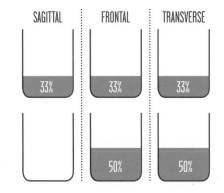

SAGITTAL	FRONTAL	TRANSVERSE
33%	33%	33%
	50%	50%

Three Cups

If a muscle is expected to operate in three dimensions of movement, then it's fair to say that one third of its potential could be apportioned to each dimension of sagittal, frontal and transverse motions. However, if a joint is limited in motion in the sagittal plane, the range of motion in a muscle is equally limited. An exchange has to happen here

in order to maintain the 100% function in the joint and the muscles attached to that joint – since that joint cannot operate at 66.6% it must demand extra work from the two remaining planes of motion. Thus we see the frontal and transverse planes of motion experiencing demands of up to 50% each to carry the burden of lack in the sagittal plane.

There is always an exchange and the outcome is always 100% or, put another way, balanced.

Tension

There is a concept in the human body called 'bio-tensegrity', which arises from the term 'tensegrity' coined by R Buckminster Fuller. The term itself is a blend of two words: 'tension' and 'integrity'. Bio-tensegrity relates the concept of tensegrity to biological entities, be it human or other animal bodies.

Tensegrity is a concept used in architecture to generate flawless stability in unstable environments, such as bridges and earthquake buildings. So what is it?

Wikipedia suggests:
"Integrity is a concept of consistency of actions, values, methods, measures, principles, expectations and outcomes."

The word 'integrity' stems from the Latin adjective *integer* (whole, complete). In this context, integrity is the inner sense of 'wholeness'.

Integrity in relation to the body then is the whole and complete approach to generating an internal consistency that optimises and manages the tension in the physical system.

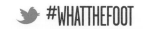

Tension is described in Wikipedia as:

"*In physics, tension is the magnitude of the pulling force exerted by a string, cable, chain or similar object on another object. It is the opposite of compression. There are two basic possibilities for systems of objects held by strings: either acceleration is zero and the system is therefore in equilibrium, or there is acceleration and therefore a net force is present. Note that a string is assumed to have negligible mass.*"

In relation to the body, we are discussing the use of muscles to exert a force on the skeletal framework — whether acting upon or reacting to the joint system. Visualise the muscles as the strings. There are two outcomes:

A) When the system is in a state of equilibrium, or centre as I have described it, the muscles are all in balance and therefore none are exerting any (or minimal) force on the skeleton. Consequently, there will be zero tension in the system.

B) As the system moves away from a state of balance, or centre, tension is increased in the string and increased forces are placed upon it, and both tension and compression are increased in the system.

Zero tension = balanced, equalised tension throughout the system

You will have seen the term 'length tension relationship' utilised in anatomy before to mean the relationship between agonist and antagonist muscles (reciprocal inhibitors). This discussion of tension integrity is a more accurate determination of tension distribution in a global system.

Zero tension

If you position the human body in neutral, all joints MUST BE in alignment and have equal access into all ranges and dimensions. All muscles MUST BE in their optimal resting state, with equal and balanced length in all muscles. Here, length tension = zero.

As we have discussed, it is impossible to hold this position since we cannot stand still. So consider what happens when the centre of mass of the skeleton moves forwards in space. Firstly, it moves away from neutral, extending the spine, creating distance between the anterior portions of the pelvis and the ribcage and externally rotating at the hip joints (providing the feet allow it). The impact on the muscles, in the anterior parts of the pelvis and spine, is for them to lengthen, in particular through the abdominals and the hip flexors — the response in these muscles is to 'stretch'. This increase in length, forged by the gapping of joints, is synonymous with an increase in tension in the muscle system. In opposition to the gapping of joints, there shall also be a closing of joints, synonymous with an increase in compression (as mentioned in the Wikipedia segment).

In equilibrium or centre, there is zero tension. As we move away from equilibrium there are increased levels of tension present in the system. Here, there must also exist compression in order to balance out the tension, thereby creating an equilibrium of sorts and thus abiding by the rule of 100% functionality as discussed earlier.

However, in an environment of perceived centre, when you are not in a state of equilibrium, there exists permanent areas of tension and permanent areas of compression in the body: each contributing

If you position the human body in neutral, all joints MUST BE in alignment and have equal access into all ranges and dimensions. All muscles MUST BE in their optimal resting state, with equal and balanced length in all muscles. Here, length tension = zero

to the downgrade in optimal function, which affects performance and lends itself to pain.

Put another way, 'permanent areas of tension' look like a series of long muscles and gapped joints, as noticed in states of poor posture and poor movement habits, naturally accompanied by shorter muscles and closed joints.

For instance, a lateral flexion in the spine changes the length tension relationship in the muscles and soft tissue that relate directly (and indirectly) to the spine. In a lateral flexion of the spine to the right, muscles lengthen on the left-hand side (increase in tension) and shorten on the right-hand side (compress) in the frontal plane.

If we give the tensioning side a score of +1 and the compressing side a score of –1, the mathematical arrangement is that each area of tension neutralises the compression, maintaining a total score of zero tension.

It's not as simple as that, of course. Let's imagine there is a compressive force on the left side of your low back with a score of –5. It's plausible that this amount of tension causes you significant pain.

It's possible that the right side of your low back has a tension score of +5 to equate the balance, but it's equally likely that the tension is distributed throughout the whole body with lots of scores to a lesser value of 1 at each joint. This is a perfect example of how a whole body reorganises itself around an area of pain. To unwind this or treat this would be a lot of work for somebody working in isolation on a joint-by-joint basis, but not so for somebody whose goal is to challenge the system

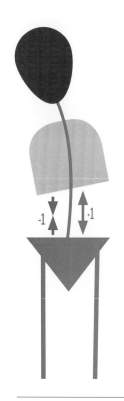

using movement to find centre anew and take a quantum leap toward zero tension, thus eliminating the physical stresses of the body.

Tension = stress

Another word for tension is stress. Stress comes in a variety of forms and whilst 'hormesis' describes that small doses of stress can be beneficial to the body, in the main the impact is negative. Tension in your body is akin to stress in your body.

Areas of compression lead to joint impingements and areas of tension lead to muscle strains and tears. Both of which you want to avoid or move away from and both of which can be alleviated and even eliminated as you bring your body back to a state of dynamic equilibrium.

Bearing all of the above in mind, if we can access zero tension and find our optimal centre then we naturally remove excess tension and compressive forces from the system and thus eliminate the stress in the body, too. This is the framework for a biomechanical quantum leap.

Big rule #5 suggests that the body is hardwired to do just that and the awareness of this pain-free and performance-enhancing state comes pre-installed in our software.

And it is... There is only one place in the body where tension is eliminated from the system — in centre. The moment the brain becomes aware of that, it is hardwired to notice that there is no longer tension or effort in the system and recognises this purely as an efficient place of rest.

Dynamically, the neutral place doesn't exist and the vibration in the system caused by the free movement around the centre point equates to a minimal amount of tension in the system. The goal of movement is not just to get from A to B, but to get from A to B as efficiently as possible. This means that the body must be able to convert this small amount of tension into greater amounts of tension in order to be able to leave centre and return back to, and pass through it, with ease.

In the process, it generates tension (big rule #1), forces a reaction in the muscle and fascia system (big rule #2), deactivates the tension using momentum through centre (no effort) and regenerates the tension in the system again on the other side. Tension is generated most when the base of support is challenged the greatest or at maximum ranges for the movement.

When the body achieves full awareness of what is possible in movement, it learns new patterns and opens up (or reopens) new neural pathways and is presented all of a sudden with choice.

Neuroskeletal programming

Neurolinguistic programming (NLP) is a method that uses language to generate new neurological pathways in the brain that help people to overcome mental and emotional inhibitions or blockages. If it works for the brain, so it must work for the body, too! This is done by recognising a series of faulty language patterns and challenging the patterns to create new, more vital patterns and pathways in which the brain can respond. It's the same for the body and for movement.

The concept NLP uses is often simply to provide a choice for the brain. This is as simple as targeting the habit that a person uses or a pattern that they regularly run, like software, whenever a given situation arises in their life. The coaching process guides them toward a new set of choices that make the initial one seem ludicrous.

Naturally, next time the situation arises again, the brain will choose a more efficient pathway, one that will create less havoc in their life and lead to a more desirable outcome. This gives them more opportunity in life as well as greater performance or output potential, in particular if this was a business client, for example.

Neuroskeletal programming (NSP) is no different. The way we walk, sit, run and exercise in our perceived centre is done in consistent, well-formed habitual patterns. Like I said originally, the hardest habit you may ever have to break!

The problem is that we walk around using our only choice. The one single way we walk is the way we walk with every step. It's a well-formed habit. There's no reason to change it as our brain has determined this way as THE way, the most functional and energy-conserving way it knows. Sadly, THE way becomes the ONLY way and choice is eliminated. The bottom line here is that, ultimately, one choice is actually no choice.

'One choice is NO choice'

Using movement as a tool offers the brain more choices — more ways of walking, more ways for muscles to function, more range for joints to access, more communication between one and all sets of joints, and more experience of what our physical system can achieve with an increased awareness

The way we walk, sit, run and exercise in our perceived centre is done in consistent, well-formed habitual patterns

When choice becomes two or more choices, the inefficient options get left behind and the body leaps into the hard-wired and pre-installed state of perfection, choosing the choices that create access only to that state

of its whole self. When choice becomes two or more choices, the inefficient options get left behind and the body leaps into the hard-wired and pre-installed state of perfection, choosing the choices that create access only to that state. The only prerequisite for this to happen, is that all causative factors and biomechanical inhibitions have to be overcome.

The big reset button is pressed and there is no need for the body to revert back to its original suboptimally performing self! Just to make sure of this, we take the big whole-body exercises that were successful in contributing to the leap and ask the client to repeat them over and over again, to have these new patterns, pathways and habits in movement cemented in the brain.

MR C: CASE STUDY

Mr C arrived at my door, seven years in pain, with a tale of a horrific contributing accident. I could only listen in disbelief and awe that this chap was even alive.

Regardless, he has pain, and the adaptations in his body will be those of a perceived centre for him and his brain – a postural adaptation that we now know to be one of several limited options where his opportunity and performance potential is hugely compromised. So what's new? I use force pressure platforms to determine the alignment of the centre of mass and foot function through the gait cycle. His scan stated that he had over 50% of his overall bodyweight passing through his right heel and approximately 15% passing through

the left heel and each forefoot. When he told me that his right ankle, knee and hip hurt, was I surprised? Absolutely not!

I recorded his gait and it became absolutely clear that Mr C had no concept of how to use his left side when either walking or standing. Either that or his perception was, for some reason, that he simply couldn't use it and the brain had formed a habit around the little story it had concocted for itself. Mr C had seen countless practitioners, had orthotics built to accommodate the leg length differences and left foot 'dysfunction' and had taken things into his own hands: time to get fit and sort things out that way – by going for a run. BOOM! There was no way his body could operate at higher speeds than limping, so the pain simply became too much. Once again, an unsolvable case had landed at my door.

In actual fact, like all the case studies in this book, Mr C was a pretty straightforward case. He couldn't use his left leg in gait (-10) and used his right leg way too much in gait and standing (+10) and his whole body was simply surviving in this way.

So I taught him to use his left leg. It's not rocket science, ladies and gentlemen! To treat the hip, knee and ankle on the right – the painful ones – was absolutely the wrong thing to be doing in this case, since every time he got off the couch and said thank you to the practitioner, he simply placed over 50% of weight through his right heel and limped right out of the door! To my mind, that is not therapy.

The images to the right show the changes in pressure distribution in Mr C's stance one hour apart – before and after the session. Mr C could not believe two things: 1) that the visual change was so significant; and 2) that he was actually out of pain. Completely.

The whole-body approach had changed the way the whole left side operated at each significant phase of the gait cycle (head to toe) in a series of simple dynamic exercises. This was all done by teaching muscles to lengthen before they contract, to mobilise the joints correctly per each gait phase, and force the appropriate reaction in the muscles, thus enhancing his overall awareness of a brand new centre. He recently informed me and thanked me for creating the opportunity for him to get back to work on a regular basis (his goal and version of performance) and was pleased to announce that he now leads a pain-free existence thanks to a series of movement-orientated exercises that I gave him. We had two sessions in total after seven years of pain.

What I actually did was give his brain two choices:
a) to walk in a way that causes no pain OR
b) to walk in a way that causes pain

Thankfully, the subconscious brain is not daft and the change was quick and powerful.

Having looked closely at the five big rules, I now think it's important to bring the rules to life in a few key areas and bring some awareness to how this physical system copes and adapts to its external environment and life as a whole.

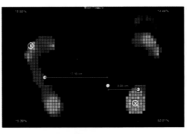

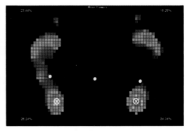

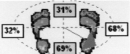

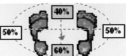

IN SUMMARY

▶ Your body knows how to position itself to overcome its inhibitions and access its most optimal state for NOW.

▶ It does this by thriving on the power of choice and new awareness of what it's not doing, that it could be doing.

▶ The body is a closed system that has the capacity to redistribute its global tension and compression relationships around the body to facilitate all movement.

▶ The brain will also self-select a posture that appears negative and yet provides support for a perceived failure in the global system.

▶ You as a practitioner cannot give someone their centre back. You must create an environment for them to find it themselves.

▶ A hard-wired state will only change if the overall value of the new state exceeds the value of the previous state. This must associate itself with a whole-body change that shifts towards effortless whilst rendering the old state effort-full.

↖ MR C CARRIED OVER HALF HIS BODYWEIGHT IN HIS RIGHT HEEL PRIOR TO THE SESSION
↑ MR C WALKED OUT IN A MUCH HIGHER STATE OF BALANCE AND PAIN FREE, WITH HIS OVERALL FIGURES READING 50%/50% (LEFT TO RIGHT) AND 60%/40% (POSTERIOR TO ANTERIOR)

PART
2

CHAPTER 4 HARDWIRED

CHAPTER 4: HARDWIRED

"When we are no longer able to change a situation, we are challenged to change ourselves."
Viktor E Frankl (1905–1997)

Can we tell the brain is hardwired to know what is optimal for its body? I mentioned John at the start of big rule #3. I met him at an exhibition in late January 2012. He painstakingly explained his physical pain and what that meant for him in his life. John's story is a perfect example of how the brain hardwires to accommodate the inhibitions and limitations in the physical system while undergoing a motion-based process to find centre anew.

I stood John on the foot scan to give me some insight into how he holds his posture and see if it made sense with the pain he was experiencing. I knew it would, and it did. Before we look at the scan, I'd like to preface it with what theoretically would be optimal: an optimal or balanced patient would bear weight equal to 25% in each quadrant, with 50%/50% distribution between the left and right foot and somewhere between 50% between the rearfoot

(heels) and forefoot or, as some research suggests, 60% in the rearfoot (heels) and 40% in the forefoot.

John's initial scan (31 January 2012)

When I met John at the corporate event, he stood on the foot-scanning machine and recorded a weight shift of 71% through the right foot, 69% of weight in his heels and 51.18% of weight in his right heel! That's over half of his bodyweight through one heel!

John had long-standing back pain and suffered from a large left L5/S1 disc prolapse compressing the S1 nerve root. He also had disc bulges at L3/4/5 with posterior annulus at L3/4. Three discs! His gait was laboured, with a significant lean to one side of his body, something he puts down to carrying a heavy bag on one shoulder. I put it down to a combination of bag carriage and physical mechanics – it should be clear for all to see that John was not in favour of putting weight through his left leg. Once again, nobody had addressed John's physical mechanics of movement to overcome his physical problems.

Three weeks later, John arrived for the first of four sessions with me. I put him on the foot scan and, again, the brain in its hard-wired state revealed not just similar, but virtually identical percentages of weight-bearing bias in his body. If anything, he had shifted forwards and right by 1%. These static stance assessments are taken over the period of one minute, which, according to literature, is ample time to get a consistent reading: now 68% in his heels, 72% in his right foot and 50.76% in his right heel alone (still carrying over half his body weight).

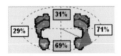

↑ JOHN'S INITIAL SCAN WHEN WE FIRST MET. IN PAIN AND UNHAPPY

106

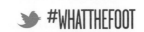

The point I would like you to take from this is his postural distribution did not change in the three weeks between these two scans (give or take 1%). Treatments he had had between the two scans had not influenced his stance or gait patterns, which ultimately would prove to be what makes the difference in John's pain and performance potential.

Before Session One (28 February 2012)

We had a movement session together. I assessed John on the force plate, both static stance assessment and in gait, as well as postural markers for alignment. I deciphered which phases of the flow motion model he was dominant in and which he was either weak in or completely unable to access. It was these particular phases and movements that I would focus on to challenge the brain as to the current perception of its hard-wired state.

Post session, I retested and, clear for all to see, John's body had moved toward centre — to my knowledge, for the first time in, most likely, years. We can see how his centre of mass has changed, which must mean his joint alignment has changed, and equally his muscle and soft tissue balance must have changed as well. He was now holding his weight with 65% in his heels, but, more importantly, 56% in his right foot with 39.15% in his right heel. We certainly weren't done, but the awareness of freedom in John's body was clear and the pain he was used to feeling was not there. Gone. It was like he was standing in a brand new body with the difference between the old and new being so stark that it actually felt pain free. His nervous system was no longer firing warning shots (experienced as pain in the brain) since the tension and compression relationships in the muscles and the joints was no longer being compromised. He was now bearing

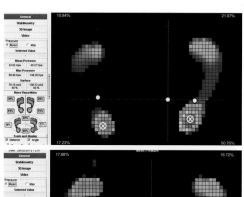

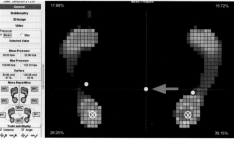

↑ TOP: PRE SESSION ONE ↑ ABOVE: POST SESSION ONE

44% of his weight through the left foot that he never used to use. This, naturally, has huge carry over to his physical wellbeing.

After Session One (28 February 2012)

The challenge now was to keep it that way. For me, that's the easy part. The patterns that John was failing to use in his daily walking — which had already contributed to the shift in the session — were to be set as his homework to remind the brain on a twice to thrice daily basis of what his body is actually capable of. I'm not talking stretches or TVA draws, or even stretch/strengthen protocol (see rants), but global physical movement patterns that replicate the phases of the flow motion model, which his brain had forgotten about over the 20 years since his injury.

Here's what happened three weeks later when he stood on the force platform again:

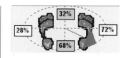

↑ PRE SESSION ONE (UNCHANGED IN THREE WEEKS)

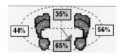

↑ POST SESSION ONE, NOTICE THE SHIFT IN HIS CENTRE OF MASS AND WEIGHT DISTRIBUTION CHANGES AFTER THE FIRST SESSION

WHAT THE FOOT?

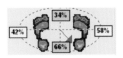

↑ PRE SESSION TWO
(UNCHANGED IN THREE WEEKS)

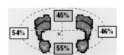

↑ ONE HOUR LATER, HIS
STANCE FAVOURS LEFT
SIDE FOR FIRST TIME IN
PROBABLY 20 YEARS

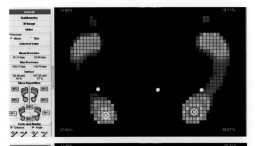

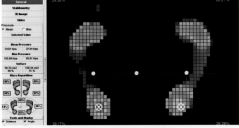

Before Session Two (22 March 2012)

Give or take a per cent or two, John was still in the same position and global posture that he held after one hours' work a month before. Yes, he had shifted a small amount back towards the right (by 2%) and slightly backwards (by 1%), but he had learnt the value of not holding weight in his right heel. With only the homework to go on, John had reduced the amount of weight he holds in his right heel from 39.15% to 38.87%. This had become possible by the apparent change in his global percentages via an increase of weight-bearing in his right forefoot instead from 16.72% to 19.11%.

Things had held after one hours' work and three weeks' homework. This was good, seeing as he had to fly to see me in London from Scotland for a session. But work was still to be done. I reassessed and continued with the programme, reassessing where his body is NOW, what shifts and changes it had made and what needed to be done today.

Certainly more movement, but, in essence, more communication with the brain to influence more optimal posture, stance and gait patterns that would prove more efficient and cause less pain. I was surprised to see what happened next.

After Session Two (22 March 2012)

John's pain had been present for 20 years. He adapted his posture as a result of the injury that occurred originally. I don't know for sure, but since he has carried the symptoms for the duration of that period, I would happily hypothesise that his posture had not shifted and changed too much in that time. It's very likely he had always carried the majority of his bodyweight in his right foot/ heel, and that bias or imbalance placed the body under significant stress due to the poor mechanical alignment and subsequent pressure on the joints and nervous system.

That's why I was surprised to discover that, after the second session, John had shifted his bodyweight onto the left side for the first time in a long time. This was the big shift. He was now holding his weight with 55% in his heels (11% less than prior to the session), remarkably 26.28% in his right foot (almost half the amount compared to six weeks earlier) and only 46% through his right foot, with 54% through his left foot compared to 29% when we started. He was now significantly using his left leg to both stand on and walk on.

Think of it like this: if you equally use both feet to stand on, the spine will stand tall; if you favour one side more than the other, the spine will lean to one side. A persistent lateral flexion of the spine will always compress the vertebral joints on one side, increasing pressure on the discs whilst increasing tension in the muscle system on the opposite side as the muscles act to decelerate further the lateral flexion of the spine. With 72% of weight through one foot, the tension and compression relationship will be significant and a more centred distribution of mass will mean less compression and less tension, which can be the difference between pain and no pain. Since John was slightly favouring the left side for the first time in years, the total body alignment was in a completely new space, which was pain free, and has set him up to get his active life back on track.

This was a classic case of a person's pain being an outcome of whole-body positioning, alignment and access to usage of the structures in place. As long as John held 70+% of his weight through the right side – how his body and brain had hardwired to determine what, for him, was the most efficient way to be – he would always struggle with pain until his overall postural alignment could be challenged in such a way that his brain deciphered a more optimal way of being, standing and walking. This can only be done by reintroducing movement patterns, which the client has avoided for years, back into the system. A joint-by-joint approach will unlikely have this outcome, since all joints are simultaneously in states of motion and feed back off each other, managed by all of the muscles, not just the ones attached to that particular joint. In order to make a shift like this, the brain and the nervous system, as well as the musculoskeletal system, must all have a new appreciation of movement that no longer creates tension and compression in the system, but allows for freedom of movement, optimal joint motion and balanced access to soft tissue, in a wholly integrated environment.

THANK YOU, GARY

Gary,

I had a great experience working with you last year to address 20 years of significant pain in my body as a direct result of a footballing injury to my lower back and ribcage. You focused on my balance and posture when everyone else focused on the pain. I remember the first time I stood on the foot plate and it registered 72% of my weight on my right foot. It seems I was overcompensating for my footballing injury by shifting my weight to attempt to reduce back pain and seemingly causing much more!

I trusted the process and put my faith in you to get me mobile and more balanced. Through a series of exercises, which I rigidly stuck to at home, my posture and balance improved and overall back pain receded. My balance is now equal and I do not suffer the pain that I previously endured. I don't do the exercises as much now, but I have replaced this with more exercise in general. I have taken a 15-month (prepaid) membership at my local golf and country club. I am going along four times a week, either to swim (including sauna and steam room), or play squash (love it) or snooker. I could never have managed this without your help and support. The weather has been against playing golf, but I am signing up to lessons with the pro once the weather gets better. It is over 10 years since I last played golf and I cannot wait to give it a go.

Thank you, Gary.
John Ellis

CHAPTER 5:
THE FORGOTTEN BODY PART

"I am everything. I am nothing. I am powerful. I am forgotten." Jennifer Lynn Barnes, *Nobody*

Student Becky: "My client has knee pain, has very obviously got no VMO (vastus medialis obliquus) muscle, and what I noticed that accompanies it is a really stiff forefoot (varus and stuck in abduction) and a really loose and wobbly rearfoot."

My response: "The varus forefoot will drive the unstable heel into a pronated position, which works up the kinetic chain to drive the knee into a valgus position due to the time it takes to get her big toe to make contact with the floor. You will find that her VMO is 'locked long' and the body finds itself in a state where it can no longer lengthen the muscle any further to give it the opportunity to contract because the stiff forefoot is dictating the length tensions in the muscle and fascial system in both stance and gait.

"My suggestion is to tackle the stiffness in the forefoot using a wedge, creating the possibility of integrated movement between the forefoot and the rearfoot so as to bring some balance to the foot itself. What you will find is there is always excess mobility somewhere when there is excess stiffness somewhere else – in a 100% functioning environment, where tension is merely exchanged on a persistent basis, this is always the case. In this case it's the forefoot and rearfoot relationship for your client.

"By increasing mobility in the forefoot, you will find that the mobility in the rearfoot changes and it will actually strengthen as the forces rebalance. You will also find that as the forefoot becomes less abducted, and more adducted and less varus and more balanced, then the timing of contact through the big toe will naturally change, thus transforming the relationship between the foot and the knee. The now less pronated foot and more stable rearfoot will mean that the VMO muscle is no longer 'locked long' and an environment has been created whereby that muscle can now lengthen to generate a contraction response and by design, as opposed to coincidence, the joints of the knee will have changed their own alignment, thus relieving any compression or tension-related pain in the joint."

The hard part of this was the diagnosis, which Becky had nailed! The easy part, once she understood the mechanics of stiffness versus mobility, was making the change. The problem here is that such a knee pain would have most fitness and therapy professionals treating the knee on a couch when, very obviously (to me at least), making a simple change in the foot would make all the difference.

Ever since I entered the health and fitness industry in 1999, I have referred to the foot as 'the forgotten body part' as nobody, but nobody, was talking about it. I think this has improved today, but my feeling is that still the industry has very little awareness of the

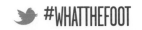

power held in the two plates of meat we spend our life on.

I love your feet

It never fails to amaze me: out of the number of practitioners I work with, very few are bold enough to say that, yes, they understand the human foot.

The foot has become the forgotten body part, the one that nobody cares about. Some yoga practitioners and physical therapists recommend stretching and some basic exercises to 'shorten' the foot to return an arch to it. Other practitioners have been taught to recognise a flat foot when they see one and promote the use of orthotics or insoles to control the foot.

I always have to ask the question, WHY would we want to control a foot that has such phenomenal mobility available to it? Would it not be better to understand the foot better, how it moves and acts, to dictate and predetermine all human movement, stance and postures?

Stand up. Ask yourself what part of your body is receiving feedback from the outside world? Your feet? Now change your stance; turn a foot in or out; place a book under one foot and notice the impact that subtle changes down there have on your whole body. Can you feel it?

As a bodyworker, it is actually your duty to discover priceless information on the human foot, to understand its role in human movement, its role in standing, its role in performance and potential, and then learn how to bring it alive in ways you never thought possible AND do all this in less than 20 minutes. You can change your client's life by giving them their foot mobility back.

Shoulder pain can be caused by inhibitions and imbalances in the feet. Back pain is never present where two perfectly articulating feet are dictating movement up the kinetic chain.

There is a reason I love your feet... because they bring the FIVE BIG RULES of human movement alive and make physical human healing a real and achievable possibility.

Complexity

One of the reasons the foot is so neglected is the sheer complexity of it. How many bones and joints? There are so many complicated muscle names and impossible-to-remember origins and insertions. I get it. However, to bring simplicity to that, when you look at the whole body, its relationship with the feet is, well, simple!

Your feet bring the FIVE BIG RULES to life

One foot has 33 joints and 26 bones. Your spine has 33 joints and 34 bones. Big rule #2 states that joints ACT and muscles REACT. Since both structures harbour 33 articulating joints, isn't the impact of movement in each of your feet, therefore, equally as important as movement in your spine?

I'll let you decide.

Firstly, there are two feet – that's 66 articulating joints impacting on the rest of the body. Secondly, the joints of the spine are linear and operate one vertebrae over the next; in the foot the joints are non-linear with some individual bones sharing several joints with other bones. The third or lateral cuneiform, for instance, has joint surfaces with six other bones.

> One foot has 33 joints and 26 bones. Your spine has 33 joints and 34 bones. Big rule #2 states that joints ACT and muscles REACT. Since both structures harbour 33 articulating joints, isn't the impact of movement in each of your feet, therefore, equally as important as movement in your spine?

WHAT THE FOOT?

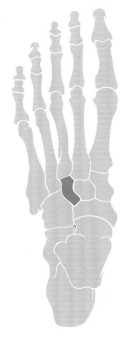

⬆ IN CONTRAST TO A VERTEBRAE, WHICH HAS A JOINT ABOVE AND BELOW, THE THIRD CUNEIFORM IS SURROUNDED BY JOINTS ON ALL SIDES

This makes it that little bit more complicated when it comes to pure mechanics of movement. Just as there are two feet, there is only one spine (don't say I never teach you anything, huh?). This means that the two feet are required to bring about balance in the skeleton above by having two feet that are fully able to articulate all 33 joints equally. Any difference between the left and right foot equals distortion up the kinetic chain.

If one foot pronates more than the other (not unusual) then there will be huge impact up the chain – for instance, exerting a rotational influence on, or an s-shape curve in, the spine.

It is not only my belief, but I also have many examples of a 'scoliosis' purely being the example of two feet that articulate differently to one another. With that in mind, it is very clear to me that the feet play a huge role in influencing the spine. Feet ACT, body REACTS? #footforthought...

The way our feet articulate is incredible and the margin for error is so small that we can define literally hundreds of pathologies for each malfunction in the foot. This is where it takes years at university to learn each pathology and how to treat it, whether manually or with orthotics.

Perfect set-up
The foot is perfectly set up for standing and mobilising our mass forwards in efficient and energy-conserving gait. It also has the capacity to adapt and downgrade its own usage in response to overall physical posture and inhibitions.

It really is a chicken and egg scenario: problems in the body will work down to the foot and problems in the foot quickly spread to the body.

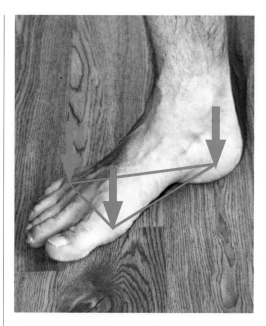

⬆ THE FOOT IS A TRIPOD

Having said that, making corrections to a body part such as a shoulder, rarely will impact on the foot, BUT making corrections to the foot function ALWAYS seems to impact on the rest of the body.

It's having this knowledge and awareness of the five big rules that makes powerful change in the workings of the human body possible.

Tripod
The foot is a tripod formed by having the heel, big toe and little toe on the floor. In this position, the foot will stand tall in what we recognise as neutral, or it will stand pronated (flatter) or supinated (high arched), all depending on the relationship between these three points of contact.

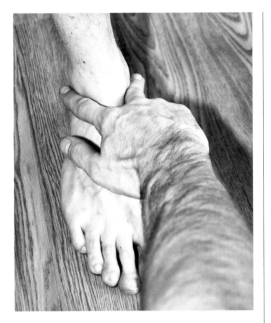

↑ TWO-FINGER TEST

Finger test

A simple test is to jam your two fingers under the ankle bones and let them come to rest, naturally. The point of the 'V' formed by the two fingers will point down the line of the second toe (neutral), medial to the second toe (pronated), or lateral to the second toe (supinated). This can be influenced and create misleading conclusions, so in order to be accurate, it helps to 'know' the foot and, of course, to practise.

The outcome of this test provides a huge amount of information about the overall posture of the body as well as highlighting a fundamental imbalance between the left and right foot. It's rare that this test will reveal balance in any one pair of feet, and where research tends to create 'norm' ranges – i.e. to

suggest that a slight imbalance is OK – what I notice is that any imbalance here reaches all the way up the body and becomes highly noticeable.

The talus bone – aka the driver of the bus

The talus bone sits beneath the tibia and fibula and forms the connection between the upper body and the foot. It's known as the 'dumb' bone because it has no muscular insertions on the bone at all.

The talus, however, is anything but dumb as it plays a huge role in dictating movement both from the body and into the foot as well as from the ground and up through the body.

I liken the talus to a head wearing headphones – the headphones being the ankle bones. When I look left, the headphones simply follow the head to the left, too. This movement of the talus dictates and drives the ankle bones and, subsequently, the whole shin and knee in the same direction.

The finger test indicates the angle that the face of the talus is pointing and thus shows you the angle of the shin and knee, and you can begin to trace this up the body. If the face of the talus moves medially (inwards), the foot pronates and the headphones/ankles follow it, resulting in a medial rotation of the shin, knee and femur. The knock-on effect through the whole body of this simple movement is enormous and virtually every practitioner on the planet is missing it – by simply not looking for it – and it goes unnoticed in assessment of your patient on the couch or in non-weight-bearing scenarios.

In this sense I describe the talus as the steering wheel or the 'driver of the bus' – our body being the bus. Where the talus goes, the whole body will follow.

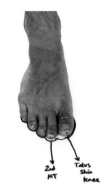

↑ AS THE TALUS BONE LOOKS LEFT TOWARDS THE BIG TOE IT CAUSES THE SHIN, KNEE AND THE WHOLE BODY TO FOLLOW IT

WHAT THE FOOT?

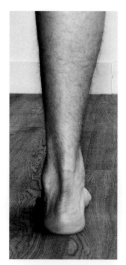

⬆ THE REARFOOT: A VERY
IMPORTANT STRUCTURE
IN THE BODY

At this point, I return to my brief point of creating norms around sub-talar joint (STJ) axis angles. The experts suggest that a norm range of 0° to 16° caters for an acceptable STJ axis. However, if one foot has a 0° axis and the other has a 16° axis, you will notice the rotational impact that this has on the whole body – a body that, now, will no longer be in balance.

The rearfoot

The rearfoot can be described as the talus and the calcaneous. It is the first part of the foot that comes into contact with the ground on walking and thus activates big rule #2. The calcaneous is forced into movement as the heel hits the ground, and muscles must react to this movement. The timing of this muscular reaction determines the overall outcome of movement in both the foot and the body from this moment until the opposite heel is next placed on the ground, one step later.

Wouldn't you agree that this makes the rearfoot a very important structure in the body?

The timing of this moment influences such things as TVA activation, glute firing potential, everything from hip flexor to shoulder function, and governs such things as knee, hip and back pain!

The rearfoot has two key joints: the ankle/talo-crural joint (TCJ) and the STJ.

To keep things simple, we can say that the ankle (TCJ) is a one-dimensional joint that operates in the sagittal plane and therefore can flex and extend only – known as dorsiflexion and plantarflexion of the ankle.

	PRONATION	SUPINATION
SAGITTAL PLANE	DORSIFLEXION	PLANTAR-FLEXION
FRONTAL PLANE	EVERSION	INVERSION
TRANSVERSE PLANE	INTERNAL ROTATION	EXTERNAL ROTATION

The STJ operates in two planes – frontal and transverse – meaning it can invert and evert as well as internally rotate and externally rotate. The magic of the rearfoot, however, is that in movement or when weight-bearing, it's impossible, thankfully, to have a complex array of movement here.

One thing you'll notice as you begin to play with the foot is that it's impossible to invert the calcaneous AND internally rotate the rearfoot at the same time. Any internal rotation will always lead directly to an eversion of the calcaneous and vice versa.

What's possible is this:

The red box above highlights that we cannot separate eversion and internal rotation in a weight-bearing rearfoot. So, when the talus rotates to the inside, it is naturally accompanied by internal rotation of the rearfoot, which must couple with eversion of the calcaneous. This causes a flattening of the foot, otherwise known as pronation.

When the talus rotates to the outside, it is accompanied by external rotation of the rearfoot, which must couple with inversion of the calcaneous – this is highlighted in the green box. This causes an increase in arch height, otherwise known as supination.

Type I and type II pronation

Since there is a possible combination of scenarios in the rearfoot, as shown in the table on the left, I have chosen to name the type of pronation (and supination) as 'type I' and 'type II'.

Type I pronation is the ideal pronation that we want to see in the stance phase of gait, and type II pronation is a type of pronation that can occur in the body, but you wouldn't necessarily want to see it present in the gait cycle, though it can be common in poor supinators or those with a weak extensor chain.

Pronation operates in the full three dimensions or planes of movement in the body.

A type I pronation is recognised when there is dorsiflexion of the ankle and eversion and internal rotation of the rearfoot or STJ, as read in the middle column of the same table. Since it is possible to fix the movement of the STJ in eversion and internal rotation AND change the position of the TCJ (ankle) from dorsiflexed to plantarflexed, we create a different type of pronated foot.

A type II pronation is recognised, then, when there is plantarflexion of the ankle accompanied by eversion and internal rotation of the rearfoot or STJ. This can be seen, for instance, when the foot flattens whilst the knee extends. Knee extension accompanies a plantarflexion of the ankle – which you definitely do not want to be present in the full weight-bearing phase of gait. This can and does happen. In actual fact, I see it a lot.

Type I and type II supination

Type I and type II supinations aren't necessarily good or bad. I have chosen to name them so purely for recognition purposes.

Type I supination is accompanied by the following three-dimensional movements: plantarflexion of the ankle as well as inversion and external rotation of the rearfoot.

Again, fixing the STJ in supination whilst sliding the ankle into dorsiflexion creates a different type of supinated foot. I call it a type II supination and is when the rearfoot inverts and externally rotates while the ankle is dorsiflexing.

Both type I and type II supination can occur at different times in the gait cycle and frequently show up in different sports, so to be able to do both is actually very important indeed for the human body. Can you access both?

The forefoot

The actions in the rearfoot as described above depend a huge amount on the timing of movement in the forefoot. The timing of the movement is reliant on one thing: the amount of time it takes the big toe to come into contact with the ground post heel strike.

The longer it takes the big toe to hit the ground, the more the foot will pronate. Most flat feet can be corrected if the timing of the big toe meeting the ground is encouraged to happen sooner.

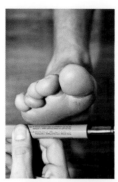

↑ THIS VARUS FOREFOOT CHANGES THE TIMINGS OF THE FOREFOOT ENTERING INTO THE GROUND AND HAS HUGE IMPACT ON OVERALL FOOT MECHANICS IN THE STANCE PHASE OF GAIT. A VARUS FOREFOOT WILL ALWAYS LEAD TO AN OVER-PRONATING FOOT IN GAIT

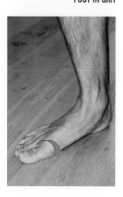

The sooner the big toe comes into contact with the ground, the higher the arch will be, to the point where if it comes into contact too quickly, it can lead to high-arched supinated feet. In this case, delaying the time it takes to bring the toe onto the ground will reduce the amount of supination and optimise the amount of pronation and supination able to take place.

If the function of the rearfoot predetermines movement through the whole body, and the rearfoot relies on the timing of the big toe to hit the ground optimally, then all of a sudden this big toe of ours becomes very important indeed!

THE GREAT HALLUX

When I was young, somebody told me that without our big toes we couldn't actually stand up! I wasn't sure at the time just how close to the truth this statement was!

Not only is the timing of the big toe important, but it has a really cool functionality to it as well – one that, most likely, is being overlooked in our assessments of people and patients.

Laid on a couch or assessing a squat, I can see how one might completely overlook the value of the big toe as a precursor for what's going on in the body. Absolutely. But once you learn the intricacies of the toe there is simply no going back.

In essence, the big toe is the starting point for the extensor chain. If the toe doesn't work, I can guarantee that the extensor chain does not work either. And no extensions, abductions or external rotations of your glutes are going to help the situation.

What about tight calves and hamstrings? Influenced by big toe function? You bet.

WINDLASS MECHANISM

The windlass mechanism was discovered by Hicks in 1954. Basically, it suggests that the big toe and the long flexor muscle that inserts onto the big toe, flexor hallucis longus (FHL), create a mechanism that has significant mechanical advantage over any other joint and muscle combination in the human body.

Quite simply, it is the most important lever in the human body. Bar none.

When you lift your big toe, you add tension into the plantar fascia and the long flexor muscles. Ideally you will see the rearfoot invert and externally rotate as well. Lifting the toe should initiate a supinatory response in the rearfoot.

Problems arise when your client cannot achieve approximately 60° of dorsiflexion (lifting off the floor) in the big toe.

Equally so, problems are always present when the big toe is lifted and the rearfoot does not invert and externally rotate.

In the image opposite, this professional footballer lifts his left toe and experiences supination of the rearfoot, but when he lifts the right toe, it highlights two problems:
a) less range in toe dorsiflexion
b) coupled with pronation in the rearfoot

Every step he takes is governed by this factor and affects his whole kinetic chain and musculoskeletal system.

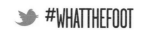

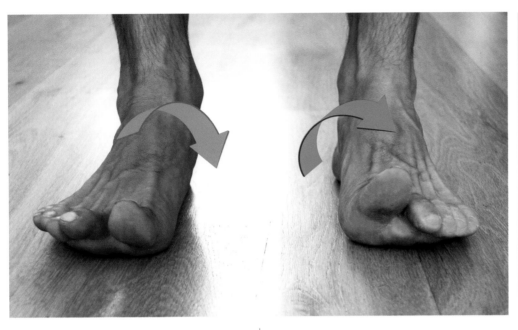

The big toe is optimised only in centre or at 60° of flexion

Some people can lift their toes way over 60° and some can't lift them at all. Neither of these create a useful outcome since 60° is optimal and fits perfectly into the model of centre.

More than 60° or less than 60° creates extensor chain limitations. The big toe is optimised only in centre or at 60° of flexion.

‹ 60°	CENTRE	› 60°
(OUCH!)	(AHHH)	(OUCH!)
☹	☺	☹

The windlass mechanism is fully active throughout the gait cycle, and inhibition in the client's ability to access it freely demands large amounts of compensation throughout the kinetic chain: such as overactive extensor digitorum longus (EDL), confused hip flexors, limited spinal extension and inhibited extensor chain muscles, such as hamstrings, glutes, piriformis and calves. More locally, however, the failure to activate the windlass mechanism normally leads to one disruptive outcome – pronated feet.

Optimal gait requires a specific role of the big toe. As I have said numerous times in the book already, when one joint fails, many joints fail. If this one fails you are on a hiding to nothing. Thankfully, it's simple enough to restore the functionality down there, without relying on orthotics as a start point.

WHAT THE FOOT?

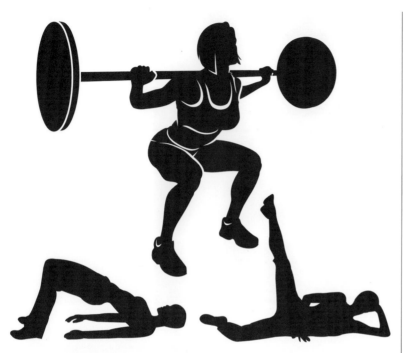

↑ CONCENTRIC ACTIONS TO STIMULATE THE GLUTES: THESE CAN BE EXAMPLES OF SHORTENING WITHOUT FULL LOAD TAKING PLACE FIRST. IN ACTUAL FACT, TO WAKE THE GLUTES UP REQUIRES A VERY DIFFERENT APPROACH WHEN RELATING THE BUTT TO THE FOOT, AND BRINGS ALIVE THE VALUE OF PRONATING THE FOOT

TURNED-OUT FEET

The old 'duck' feet or '10 to two' feet have become a mainstay of human anatomy, I'm sad to say. You know when you walk along the beach and take a look behind you at your footprints and wonder who the hell left those prints behind? It looks like you're following in the footsteps of the yeti!

Turned-out feet are yet another wonderful indicator of foot and hip function. Big rule #1 states that muscles always lengthen before they contract in movement. This means that to set itself up perfectly for gait, the brain must place the foot in a position that creates the possibility for the muscles of the foot to lengthen in order to get some reaction in the extensor chain – a contraction

that will propel us forward. The big muscles in the extensor chain, so often affected by turned-out feet, are the mighty glutes.

A QUICK LOOK AT THE GLUTES ACCORDING TO BIG RULE #1

This gives us the opportunity to take a look at how the glutes are set up to decelerate movement not just in the hip, but in the feet as well, and give you a broader look at the impact of a single muscle on a wider canvas.

The concentric actions of the glutes are:
- hip extension
- hip abduction
- hip external rotation

Unsurprisingly, you can all think of a whole host of exercises that create that environment for the glutes: squats, clams, external rotations, etc.

When the foot is in a type I pronation, as mentioned above, it is:
- dorsiflexed (TCJ)
- everted (STJ)
- internally rotated (STJ)

The driver of the bus subsequently triggers movement in the tibia, femur and pelvis, pushing them all in the same direction. In a bilateral or static stance, i.e. hip width apart, the impact of this movement at the hip, as a direct result of pronation, will be:
- hip flexion
- hip adduction and
- hip internal rotation

The exact opposite of the concentric action of the glutes!

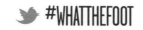

WHAT THE FOOT?

Big rule #1 states that muscles lengthen before they contract, so, in this position of hip flexion, adduction and internal rotation, the glutes are lengthened and therefore put in a position with no ensuing action but to contract. Since also joints ACT and muscles REACT, it follows that pronation of the foot creates the skeletal ACTION that generates the necessary muscle REACTION at the hip. Thus, without pronation, the glutes cannot fire.

The big butt muscles are therefore set up to decelerate:
- hip flexion
- hip adduction
- hip internal rotation
AND
- pronation of the foot...

...whilst also being responsible for generating the necessary extension at the hip. In fact, extension at the hip is wholly reliant on pronation at the foot.

Perhaps I should say that again? But louder?

"Extension at the hip is wholly reliant on pronation at the foot."

In gait, it's slightly different since the pelvis is directly influenced by the internal rotation of the talus bone. The pelvis moves away from the pronating foot in the transverse plane, leaving us ordinarily with an externally rotated hip.

The pronation in the foot in gait, then, impacts directly on the hip joint – flexing and adducting the hip, with minimal amounts of rotation taking place as the pelvis is forced to move along with the femur in line with the talus bone.

So, when the foot pronates, the hip joint (ilio-femoral joint) flexes and adducts. Both of these movements cause the glutes (as well as lateral hamstrings, VMO and calves – all extensor chain muscles) to LENGTHEN as the muscle is forced, again, into its lengthened eccentric state.

The glutes now have a role to play, which is to decelerate the movement at the hip joint – the pronating foot has put the hip joint into motion and the muscles of the hip must now act secondarily to decelerate and control that initial movement in accordance with big rule #2 – joints ACT, muscles REACT.

As the glute overcomes the movement, it shortens concentrically to bring the joint back into alignment and through to the shortened concentric phase of its movement.

Consequently, you can see that the glute will now extend and abduct the hip joint from its most flexed, adducted and neutrally rotated position (the internal rotation of the hip, for those of you who are following this, actually takes place at a slightly later phase of gait, highlighting that the full three dimensions of glute action occur at different stages in the gait cycle – so, in actual fact, to train the glute to fire in all three planes at once is squat specific, but not specific to gait).

In summary, what happened here is that the foot pronates, impacts on the hip joint and demands a response from the big butt muscles.

In order:
Pronation ➡ hip motion ➡ muscular reaction

Extension at the hip is wholly reliant on pronation at the foot

WHAT THE FOOT?

The foot pronates, impacts on the hip joint and demands a response from the big butt muscles

Joints first, muscles second.

It is this critical moment in gait that gives our extensor chain a role in locomotion. If you cannot pronate your foot, then you cannot activate your glutes.

Whenever I ask my students to name the number one sleepy muscle in the body, they always, always, say "the glutes", without exception. We have strength and conditioning coaches being handed patients from the physio with strict orders to work the glutes concentrically in a bid to switch them on.

I want to reiterate here, guys, that NO amount of extensions and external rotations will get the glutes to WAKE UP if you do not deal with the pronation issues in the foot first, since the body requires the foot to do its thing if the glutes are going to be involved in the game.

Why do all trainers and therapists report the glutes as the number one sleepy muscle in the body? Because up to 95% of people on the planet over-pronate feet in gait, and as a result can't further pronate their feet sufficiently enough to cause the reaction we want. (See page 130 of this document for reference.)

Weak glutes? Tight calves? Hamstring problems? — think feet and big toe!
#whatthefoot

Thankfully, we have set up a process at AiM that teaches you to recognise not just this coupled relationship between foot and hip, but all the possible coupled relationships in the body that

are affecting you, your clients and everybody else in the world. What's more, it's so simple once you begin looking in the right places, i.e. on the other side of the coin.

Dysfunctional?
This glute activation principle is an example of three things:

- Firstly, of how we can give a muscle NO OPTION BUT TO CONTRACT by loading it eccentrically first.
- Secondly, of how we can see just how important the integration of other body parts are to the activation of any isolated muscle.
- And thirdly, of how the body sets itself up in a way to maximise movement of any kind.

Currently, it could be deemed dysfunctional, in the example of inactive glutes, when it's actually a demonstration of pure functionality in an amazing and complex bodily system. If the feet don't work, the glutes simply downgrade their performance as they are no longer needed to decelerate a foot that is over-pronated and no longer moving at all.

BACK TO TURNED-OUT FEET

So with that in mind, do you now know why people turn their feet out to aid walking? Please allow me to tell you.

Turned-out feet are reserved for flat-footed or over-pronated people — people whose glutes aren't firing on all cylinders — and it's a way of their body screaming at you, the practitioner, something like: "Excuse me, please can you help me and WAKE MY ASS UP!?"

The body always carries hidden messages and can give you, a future connoisseur of human

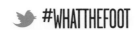

movement, the answers you seek to get to the bottom of unsolvable physical problems.

The subconscious body has made a simple adaptation to foot alignment in order to optimise its performance:

- The over-pronated foot becomes less and less pronated the more turned out it is.
- The less pronated the foot is, the more it can move into pronation.
- The more it can move into pronation, the more impact it has on the glutes eccentrically to engage them in walking and propulsion through the gait cycle.
- Turned-out feet turn the glutes on by accessing greater movement into pronation.

Our conventional approach could be to:

- consciously straighten the feet up – this never works
- apply some orthotics to minimise the over-pronation to engage the glutes – glutes will only activate if there is flexibility in the arch of the orthotic and movement is promoted
- activate the glutes through concentric training principles from neutral to extended, abducted and/or externally rotated – this is limited as the actual role of the glute is never, ever challenged

The solution to this problem is not to place the foot and hip in neutral, but to create an environment where the feet mobilise the hip in such a way that the muscles of the hip and extensor chain are challenged to eccentrically decelerate movement in the lower limbs, isometrically stabilise the movement and concentrically propel us into extension in one simple action. My advice would be that to pronate the feet more is to trigger a supinatory, extension-orientated reaction in the extensor chain.

Normally, to suggest this to educated people in the industry is to have myself laughed out of the room. Yet when we use this principle live with people from all walks of life – from the elite sportsperson to the little old lady or young child – very simply, it works every time.

WTF?

Pronation and supination

You fit somewhere along this spectrum:

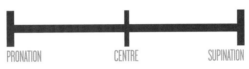

PRONATION   CENTRE   SUPINATION

Your foot has a duty to experience full pronation and full supination within optimum timings so as to generate an optimal and flowing gait cycle and release tension and inhibition in the body. Your feet are the interface between your internal and external environments and thus the state of your body depends wholly upon their ability to do just that.

As with all the movement-orientated concepts, it's important to understand that these movements (pronation and supination) exist for a reason and carry a very specific purpose and role in the human body.

CENTRE

In the diagram above, centre is the midpoint between supination and pronation; it represents neutral in the foot, which forms the perfect tripod for stance. If we focus on neutralising the foot, be it with exercise

"Excuse me, please can you help me and WAKE MY ASS UP!?"

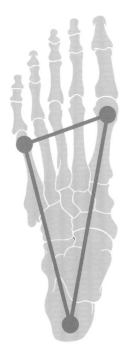

⬆ THE FOOT IS A TRIPOD WITH THREE POINTS ON THE GROUND. BETWEEN EACH POINT WE CAN SEE THREE ARCHES: MEDIAL, LATERAL AND TRANSVERSE

or orthotics, then we are failing to explore the areas around the centre point and can only offer minimal solutions to the foot and for the body. You should now also be in a position to see how this approach negatively affects glute and extensor chain function as well.

NEUTRAL

The foot in neutral is a perfect tripod, with three points on the ground. The heel, the big toe (1st metatarsal head) and the little toe (5th metatarsal head).

There are three arches:
● Medial – the one you all know about
● Lateral – the one that some of you might know about
● Transverse – the one that many of you probably don't know about. I've got news for you – it's not that important!*

What is important is being able to recognise where neutral is, how to assess whether the foot can access it or not and whether the joints can articulate through neutral so that when you look at its movement you can see whether the foot is doing what it should or not.

www.whatthefoot.co.uk/findingneutral

Outside of neutral, the foot is described as pronating to the medial side and supinating to the lateral side.

There is always an exchange in the body:
● Too much pronation means insufficient supination.
● Too much supination limits access into pronation.
● Optimal movement accesses both pronation and supination whilst passing through the centre point.

PRONATION — MOBILE ADAPTOR

Pronation is when the medial arch of the foot flattens, the joints in the foot open on the medial side and the foot spreads out to adapt dynamically to any surface it is placed upon.

As discussed above, pronation occurs at the ankle and STJ, leading to two types of pronation – I have named them 'type I' and 'type II' pronation (see page 115).

Pronation occurs to absorb the shock of ground reaction; the foot becomes flexible and mobile so as to adapt to the earth below it, whether concrete, sand or rubble, and is thus known as a mobile adaptor.

Pronation is also the moment where the muscles prepare for propulsion. The foot was designed to function on the earth and on uneven surfaces: shoes, flat level ground and concrete are its worst enemy. It gets lazy and subsequently downgrades its function, with the true role of the foot no longer needed in the flat world we have created.

Sadly, a foot lacking in functionality means potential pain for your body, regardless of the surface you live on.

---

*Some of you will pipe up at this point, knowing the importance of the transverse arch. I accept that. However, my point is simply that when you understand the movement of the foot and its connection to the whole chain, you will see transverse arches come back to life once you begin to promote movement and communication from the foot through the whole body, instead of attempting to control and stabilise it.

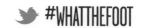

Nasty, evil pronation

Influenced by society and media, you probably recognise pronation as 'evil', something to be controlled or supported in the body. You may have heard over-pronated feet judged as being a 'flat foot' – even when it's not! You might advise unnecessary insoles in the footwear to influence it or, even worse, anti-pronation shoes! Quickly cast your mind back to the glutes and extensor chain discussion and reflect on what anti-pronation really means for these muscles. Nothing good.

Pronation is not a bad thing, but a necessary thing; if we can recognise that an over-pronating foot is the body's way of subconsciously reorganising itself to access maximal function of the body as a whole (see 'Turned-out feet' again – page 118), we can view it differently and offer it a realistic solution that encourages long-term change in the foot as opposed to a short-term intervention that will likely cause more problems down the line.

ANTI-PRONATION

The very word 'anti-pronation' makes my blood curdle!

Pronation is actually the driving force for all movement in the body. How on earth can we view it as bad when this is truly the case?

At worst, pronation can be described as a wayward movement – a deviation from where the foot wants to be, a distraction from its centre.

Yet to balance that thought, pronation is required to naturally explore our base of support, giving awareness to the muscles of the body as we orbit around our centre point.

Pronation is only a problem when we get stuck in it and can't get out of it – even then, seeking to control it is not a long-term solution. We have to promote movement in this part of our body.

Pronation initiates big rule #2. In pronation, the joint system via the calcaneous, talus and medial arch connections moves towards the ground, flattening the arch. This motion must be decelerated and controlled by the surrounding musculature to both allow and minimise the pronation – notice that to both minimise and allow is to experience optimal movement.

In pronation, the bones of the foot enter into a position that gives the muscles no option but to powerfully contract back using a supination motion, to deliver optimum movement through the foot. In this situation, muscles are lengthened first and contracted second to control and mobilise the foot and the whole body (big rule #1). An in-depth analysis into all muscles of the foot in motion shows just how many of them are lengthened during the pronation action of the foot: most all of them are perfectly set up to decelerate that pronation, driving supination, extension and locomotion via a combination of the first three big rules of movement.

Pronation has a direct impact on the centre of mass. It drives it away, pushing it towards the other foot where, hopefully, a pronation in response will knock it back, like a simple game of 'centre of mass tennis'.

When we are walking, it carries the same purpose: to stimulate muscle reaction and drive the centre of mass optimally forward, passing it from left foot to right foot and back again.

> *Pronation is only a problem when we get stuck in it*

WHAT THE FOOT?

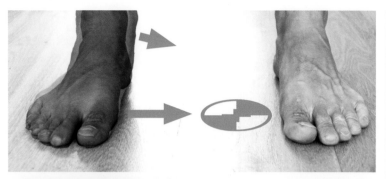

⬆ IMPACT OF A STANCE PRONATION ON THE CENTRE OF MASS

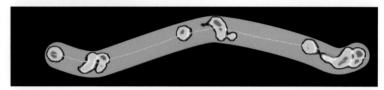

⬆ IMPACT OF DYNAMIC GAIT ON THE CENTRE OF MASS: THE WHITE LINE IN THIS DYNAMIC IMAGE IS THE CENTRE OF PRESSURE, WHICH DANCES WITH THE CENTRE OF MASS, AS I'LL EXPLAIN LATER. IN THIS IMAGE, YOU CAN EFFECTIVELY SEE HOW THE CENTRE OF MASS IS PASSED FROM ONE FOOT TO THE OTHER VIA THE EVER-ADAPTING BASE OF SUPPORT, IN THE NAME OF FORWARD LOCOMOTION AND BALANCE, OR MASS MANAGEMENT

Pronation is one of the movements in the body that enable us to mobilise the centre of mass to challenge the boundaries of our base of support and explore and challenge our physical comfort zone.

When one foot pronates more than the other, or holds a resting position that is more pronated than the other, then our centre of mass must change position.

When the centre of mass moves away from the foot that is more pronated, it changes the whole skeletal structure, and consequent global muscle tensions are altered (big rule #3).

In gait, over-pronating feet drive the centre of mass away too quickly, placing a huge demand on the muscle and fascial system to control this wayward movement. The body naturally adapts to this, so as to minimise stress on the body and downgrade overall functionality, and self-selects a new state of perceived centre in its daily quest to fulfil its goals with maximally efficient and functional movement patterns.

SIMPLE ADAPTATION TO PRONATION IN THE JOINT SYSTEM

When both feet are flat or hold a pronated position in stance, your centre of mass moves away from centre, acting directly to change alignment in the whole musculoskeletal system.

The following key muscles react by lengthening to decelerate or control this over-pronation:

- gastrocnemius
- soleus
- biceps femoris
- vastus medialis
- TFL and ITB
- glutes
- latissimus dorsi
- rhomboids
- neck flexors

To have all of these muscles in a lengthened state simply won't work for the body, thus it self-optimises for efficient movement by means of TOTAL postural adaptation.

In the case of the turned-out feet mentioned earlier in this chapter, we have seen an adaptation in the body to having excess pronation in the feet.

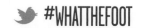

WHAT THE FOOT?

Commonly, we might ask a patient to straighten the feet up or to stretch the buttocks to encourage the feet to point straight forward – however, this approach is futile unless we can convince the body of another way to experience overall efficient movement.

This can only be done by re-educating the foot and pressing the big reset button on the body to have it operate optimally through centre.

A turned-out foot always presents itself as an internally rotated rearfoot with an external hip rotation (duck feet) and, more often than not, an anterior displacement of the centre of mass – if the weight is predominantly in the forefeet. The implications of this are huge and the potential problems that could arise are numerous, from back pain to hip pain and foot pain to neck or shoulder pain.

To teach these three integrative factors (hip, ankle and centre of mass) to communicate better and thus 'hold hands', as opposed to each of them pulling in different directions, is synonymous with creating a transformation in full-body awareness for the brain.

I present it with a new choice:
"Would the body prefer to remain turned out in the feet and hip with a pronated STJ and displaced centre of mass OR would it prefer to have the feet turned in with full ability to pronate and supinate whilst positively influencing the hips and centre of mass?"

Providing the brain with two possibilities instead of one means it can effectively choose the one it likes most.

The brain seeks balance and homeostasis, nothing more, nothing less, and thus chooses the pathway which, first and foremost, removes tension and unnecessary effort from the system. When the foot does the 'right' thing at the 'right' time in terms of gait, then flow is restored to the body. If the timing is out, it's all out. More on that a little later.

When over-pronation changes the joint system for the worse, the gait cycle and free movement are affected. Our centre of mass is incorrectly influenced and the body downgrades its output in favour of a simpler optimisation to balance out the effort required irrespective of the consequences.

SIMPLE ADAPTATION TO PRONATION IN THE MUSCLE SYSTEM

Have a look at the muscle list again. How often do you spend your time stretching or foam rolling your calves, hamstrings, glutes, TFL and ITB before or after a training session?

Here's something to consider: if your feet are flatter than they should be, it could be that you are spending that time stretching already long and tight muscles. Uh oh! Time-wasting activity alert!

That's the equivalent of Tim Ferris's 4,000,000-hour body – you will never get the result you crave, my friend.

Muscles that are too long in their resting state always feel tight as they perpetually maintain effort in an attempt to bring the body back to centre. A long muscle wants to shorten – it has to in order to normalise!

Tightness is simply the persistent isometric state of a muscle under tension. A long muscle wants to

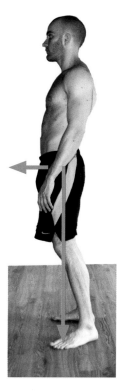

↑ FEET TURNED OUT CAN LEAD TO AN ANTERIOR DISPLACEMENT OF CENTRE OF MASS, AND THUS PELVIS, AS THE BODYWEIGHT SHIFTS IN TO THE FOREFOOT

"The ability to choose is real power." (Tim Ferris, The 4-hour Work Week)

> *Without pronation, there is nothing to slow down, and therefore no response in the muscle system*

shorten to restore balance and a short muscle wants to lengthen to restore balance.

However, since in the case of an over-pronated stance posture, all extensor muscles have lengthened and the opportunity to contract and return never arises so they all must remain long for the time being.

Why? Because it's unlikely that the body will choose to subconsciously worsen its posture in order to create more length in already long muscles to stimulate the desired reaction.

Remember that any adaptation represents a slide down the bell curve for muscle force and output potential, not to mention joint range of motion capabilities, too. To not be centred is to remain imbalanced and underutilised.

Pronation in your foot is designed to force your muscles to react and shorten (big rule #1 and #2 combined). This proves to be healthy when the muscles can pull the foot out of pronation, but unhealthy if the muscles become 'set' in this pronated position.

STATIC AND DYNAMIC PRONATION

A static pronation (flat foot) is not an ideal scenario since movement is either removed or extremely limited. A dynamic pronation is healthy as it creates a lengthening of muscles, which in turn can pull the body out of the position and back towards a centred state (big rule #1).

Pronation is neither good nor bad – it's just something that the body does and, in many cases, simply needs to do better. You can imagine its

school report card: All the potential in the world, but just not using it... I think I've heard that before somewhere!

Muscles work in an on-off-on-off environment, static only at the point between on and off. Thus the body needs to have, and indeed does have, a system that can represent an extreme of this statement: maximum extension and maximum flexion or maximum pronation and maximum supination – with the static point occurring at the maximum end range with momentum or flow carrying us from one extreme to the other in an effortless environment.

The muscles' job is to slow down the movement so as to be optimal for locomotion or the goal-driven task at hand. Without pronation, there is nothing to slow down, and therefore no response in the muscle system. So without pronation we can't have supination and without these two extremes of movement there can be no centre and no neutral position. Thus the optimisation of this central or neutral position arises purely and simply out of the awareness of, and the ability to access, the two extremes in any three-dimensional movement.

When joint motion is lacking, the muscles fail to be stimulated and in response to that they do nothing or the bare minimal. Just like you and me – without a stimulus to kick me into action I, too, would do nothing... thank goodness for my wife!

To train the body to be in neutral eliminates stimulation of any muscle. It shortens our range and minimises our potential. Many people who are gym goers or athletes become really strong

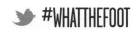

in a shortened range when naturally the goal should be to get strong in increased ranges and maximise their opportunity in their chosen sport, simultaneously minimising the risk of injury.

When I take the foot through its whole movement spectrum, the response in the WHOLE body is incredible.

The whole body reacts to the foot. It is the interface between us and the outside world when we are in an upright position – nothing else is in contact with the physical outside world.

A change in one foot creates an adaptation in the other. A change in the foot alters the impact on the centre of mass (for better or worse). A change in one foot has the power to bring the whole muscle system alive, reactivating the extensor muscles described above and eliminating that excess tension in the system. A change in the feet actually creates the healing environment we are seeking.

GRAVITY

One more thing about pronation that I think is key to understanding movement, and may help to realise that what we think we know about muscles could be limited, is this:

There is no such thing as a muscle of pronation when in an upright position.

Pronation incorporates dorsiflexion, eversion and internal rotation whilst supination incorporates plantarflexion, inversion and external rotation. If the muscles of pronation don't pronate the foot, then, firstly, what does pronate the foot and, secondly, what do the muscles of pronation do?

No muscles pronate the foot – gravity does that.

If I want to collapse my arch to the floor I simply switch off the tension in my arch and allow the foot to flatten. I can also move my pelvis to the left, flattening my right foot, or rotate my spine and pelvis to the left, also flattening the right foot – no muscles involved! Moreover, the muscles are all placed into a lengthening of some sort. I can also transfer my weight to one leg and the foot will flatten and spread again. None of these actions required me to consciously activate muscles to concentrically pronate the foot. Got that? Stand up and run through those movements I just described for yourself.

When the foot pronates, virtually all of the muscles of the foot lengthen and if big rule #1 stands true, as I believe, then that makes virtually all of the muscles 'resupinators' of the foot.

To influence the feet by accessing more pronation so as to trigger the necessary activation of the supinatory muscles and extensor chain means that the whole body begins to adapt, finding its own efficient pathways for effortless movement, incorporating both pronation and supination. Effortless movement arises when pronation and supination are equally useful and have an optimal relationship with each other, given the influence of each movement on the centre of mass.

SUPINATION – RIGID LEVER

Supination is when the medial arch increases in height, the joints in the foot close and the foot forms a rigid lever – perfect for propulsion and powering the body forwards in motion. Supination is the culmination of three-dimensional movement

The optimisation of centre arises purely and simply out of the awareness of the two extremes in any three-dimensional movement

WHAT THE FOOT?

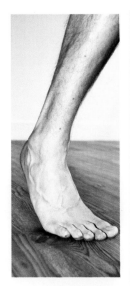

↑ SUPINATION FORMS A RIGID LEVER IN THE FOOT TO GENERATE FORWARDS PROPULSION IN MOTION

– plantarflexion, inversion and external rotation – and is measured about the STJ.

The muscles of supination, as mentioned above, are preloaded in the pronation phase, and the bones of the foot should return from their mobile adaptive state to become a rigid lever, a structure that is solid, fixed, rigid and can support the weight of the whole body for toe off or propulsion. Hint: you should access supination and the rigid lever state when you enter into a tiptoe.

You probably know concentric-based exercises that strengthen the supination muscles, such as scrunching a towel under your toes (useless) or any movement designed to shorten the foot (interesting, but could do better). The mere fact that our industry is hugely focused on the neutral position of the foot means that you may regard supination as mostly insignificant, in the same way you may have previously regarded pronation as evil.

As previously mentioned, all muscles of the foot would appear to play a major role in decelerating pronation. Thus any supination of the foot as a corrective exercise is simply a concentric shortening of the muscles of the foot.

Since the muscles 'learn' by lengthening first, supination alone is insufficient to re-educate optimal supination. So we must turn our attention to another word...

'Resupination' – the act of getting the foot back out of pronation.

RESUPINATION

I'd like to forget about the term 'supination' and focus purely on the term 'resupination'. Purely and simply, it's what millions of feet in this world are lacking.

"Normal foot types comprise around 30% of the total foot shape types within the general population. The pronator and supinator types together represent abnormal foot shape types, and account for 70% of foot shapes within the general population. The table below identifies the main differences between these two abnormal foot types."

Main Features	Pronator	Supinator
% of all abnormal foot types (70% of all foot types)	95%	5%

(www.root2being.com/the-three-foot-shapes.aspx)

The above table is clear for all to see: out of the 70% of people who have foot deformities, 95% of those people will have flat, pronated or even over-pronated feet, whilst 5% of people have high-arched feet.

That's 67% of the population who are stuck in pronation. Since pronation and supination are two sides of the movement see-saw, this means that 67% of people most likely struggle to resupinate from the pronated position. It's not anti-pronation we seek, it's a resupination to rebalance the over-pronation.

Haile Gebrselassie has HUGE over-pronation and, thankfully, HUGE resupination to make him the world's best-ever long-distance runner.

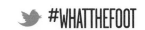

Interestingly, the 5% of supinators out there also struggle to pronate their feet, despite it being the role of gravity. This also means that they don't get the benefits of resupination either, since the muscles of supination are locked in short positions and fail to lengthen during the natural stretch phase of pronation. If they don't pronate, they don't need to resupinate!

Back to the central theme: I mentioned that once the 2nd cuneiform bone strays away from its optimal centre position, we enter a world of pathology and chaos. With 67% of people stuck in pronation, this means that the possibility of pathology is present in that portion of the population.

The report suggests that 30% of people have normal feet. Let me be clear here that I have rarely seen the 'normal' foot. Perhaps these normal-footed people don't come to my clinic. That would make sense, but being the body nerd that I am, I literally watch people all day long, in town, on the beach... I fascinate about footwear (not in the way my wife does, but at the mess it makes of our feet), I watch the influence the feet have on anybody in my vicinity. Right now there is a lady limping across the coffee shop floor. I bet two things: 1) she doesn't know she's limping; and 2) her feet function differently from each other.

A simple re-education of her body encouraging the foot to resupinate from a pronated position — by lengthening the muscles first — would create the awareness in the brain of the value of both pronation and resupination and would lend itself to relocating the 2nd cuneiform back in its ideal position. In many cases, a flat pronated foot simply needs pronating more to further lengthen the muscles and generate

a resupination awareness in that foot. Counter-logical I know. Welcome to the world of movement.

If I was to hazard a guess, having worked with athletes, friends and clients as well as both 'fit and healthy students', I don't think I have ever seen a normal foot in that population, so the figure of normal feet is probably closer to 0% than 30% if we are to call a foot normal when it operates closer to centre and freely moves either side of centre in pronation and resupination.

At this point I'd like to rewrite the pretext for the previous table:
"With virtually no normal foot types in the general population. The pronator and supinator types together represent virtually all abnormal foot shape types, and account for close to 100% of foot shapes within the general population — let's be kind and base it on 95% of the population having abnormal (non-centred) foot shapes. The table below identifies the main differences between these two abnormal foot types."

Main Features	Pronator	Supinator
% of all abnormal foot types (95% of all foot types)	95%	5%

Basically, everybody!

What is worse; since a pronated foot does not move correctly and a supinated foot does not move correctly, we're closer to the truth being that 100% of people cannot pronate their feet correctly. NOBODY.

> We're closer to the truth that actually 100% of people cannot pronate their feet correctly

WHAT THE FOOT?

To be stuck either side of centre is a problem for the body. I always suggest to students, in particular the personal trainers and yoga teachers, that instead of going to university to learn the thousands of pathologies, why not focus on the one way to get the body back to centre and eliminate the possibility of pathology – through movement.

You see, for feet to be normal, they would have to be normal in both static and dynamic function. I have seen the perfect foot, praised it even (to myself, of course), only to discover that it is locked in its neutral position, immobile and consequently the cause of all problems in the patient's body.

The other foot will always be pronated, of course, because the static neutral foot will keep the centre of mass closer to it, having lost the ability to propel

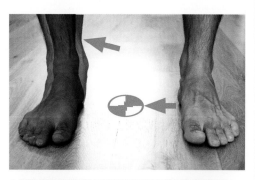

⬆ SUPINATION OF THE RIGHT FOOT BRINGS THE COFM BACK TOWARDS IT

it across to the other foot – which, of course, is one of the roles of pronation as discussed earlier – resulting in the other foot having to take on a posture that mimics pushing it away, thus pronated.

Whereas we said that pronation drives the centre of mass away from it (page 124), we can deduce that

supination or resupination brings the centre of mass back towards the foot. Resupination is also the precursor for efficient and strong forward movement of our mass due to its powerful propulsive properties.

For feet to be normal, they also have to be identical since a single degree of difference in the sub-talar axis will create movement up the chain in one direction. It has been suggested that a 'normal' STJ axis can be up to 16°.

Is this normal?
● Left STJ axis = neutral
● Right STJ axis = 10°

The outcome in the whole body here will be internally rotated right leg relative to the neutral left with a left rotated pelvis and counterrotation in the spine.
● Normal? No
● Causative of imbalance? Yes

SIMPLE ADAPTATION TO SUPINATION IN THE JOINT SYSTEM

A high-arched rigid foot limits hugely the potential in the joint system. There tends to be little or no influence up the kinetic chain in comparison to the pronating foot. Noticeably, the legs become externally rotated and the pelvis tends to access more rotation than anything else.

Since the foot does not drive the centre of mass away from it, there tends to be a shorter stride and less exploration of the base of support – a direct consequence of this is that muscles aren't stimulated in the way we have previously described, since all muscles respond to pronation… Limited joint action means limited muscular response and similar physical problems. Someone with supinated feet might describe or present with incredible stiffness.

SIMPLE ADAPTATION TO SUPINATION IN THE MUSCLE SYSTEM

There will be no or little internal rotation and the extensor chain muscles of the glutes, hamstrings and calves will find themselves in a shortened state – appearing as if to be overworking to prevent any pronation at all.

Where the muscles are tight and long in an over-pronated foot, the muscles are tight and short in a rigid supinated foot. Yet in both scenarios movement is not present and the two cases are equally as bad as each other.

I hope it's clear that for the foot to self-optimise its role in both static stance and dynamic gait, it needs a full experience of both pronation and supination through centre and to be equally utilised in both feet.

When you learn to generate that movement and link it up to the higher joints, aka knee, hips, spine, etc, it is possible to readjust and re-educate the whole body in a very short time frame. The brain knows where it wants to be – it just needs better choices and to be taught how to override old habitual patterns.

COUPLING

I suggested earlier in the book that there are only a handful of postural anomalies in the body. They all lead to changes in the alignment and functionality of the feet. Whether the chicken or the egg came first, it does not matter, for a simple change in the mechanics of the foot will always have a dramatic impact on the rest of the body.

If the foundations of your house move, you would know about it. Wouldn't you?

One of the postural anomalies that rarely walks in your door is the hyper-extended spine. Put simply, the body equates spinal extension not with supination, but with resupination. If your feet cannot resupinate from a pronated position you will not be able to effectively extend your spine.

The spine extends twice per gait cycle: once when the left foot is flat on the ground and once when the right foot is flat on the ground. If it cannot extend, then the timing of foot contact with the ground will be poor, most likely over-pronating (95%), and its subsequent failure to resupinate means the extension of the spine becomes nigh on impossible. Equally so, the supinated high-arched foot (5%) fails to stimulate the extensor chain and thus spinal extension in gait is impossible.

The same can be said of hip extension: if your feet cannot resupinate from a pronated position you will not be able to extend your hips. The downside of this is that the posterior muscles of the back, butt and legs are unable to fully contract to engage full locomotion.

Having watched probably thousands of people walk, I estimate that more than nine out of 10 people fail to extend their hips and spine in gait. This is potentially due to the fact that the majority of people are either over-pronated or over-supinated and they tend to compensate by flexing the hip flexors to lift the leg forward, instead of lengthening them first to create free motion forwards. The latter is effortless, the former requires effort and whole-body adaptation or compensation. The inability to extend our spine further reduces our ability to extend or lengthen the

If your feet cannot resupinate from a pronated position you will not be able to effectively extend your spine

*Flexion + more
flexion = Flexion!*

abdominal muscles, so they, too, are operating in a suboptimal environment. Any wonder the 'six-pack abs' dream is so prevalent?

FLEXION AND YOUR SIX-PACK HUNT

In a flexed-up world, we sit down all day, walk around staring down at our phones, driving our cars, walking with flexed hips, flexed spine and pronated feet, and rarely get the opportunity to stand tall. Our natural response to this is the desire for a flatter tummy and a six-pack.

This type of postural slump has huge knock-on effects: it causes the belly to pop out and appear unsightly, effectively deactivating the abdominal muscles (even before we look at nutrition and hormonal imbalance, poor posture inhibits your flat-stomach potential). How do we deal with this? Sit-ups.

Please... Really? More flexion?

Sit-ups never have and never will be effective in an environment where you spend your day in flexion.

Flexion + more flexion = Flexion!

This posture – our natural adaptation to life – shortens the flexor muscles and lengthens the extensor muscles. Think of it like this: the extensor muscles in the back lengthen in preparation for the day you finally decide to stand up tall, so that when you do they can contract back to upright – they lengthen first to create an environment for extension second.

The problem is, the longer you take to do this, the more stuck and habit-formed the muscles become

and we quickly adapt to a new perceived centre and consequent downgrade in potential.

Whereas conventional wisdom suggests flexing your flexors (abs, biceps, pecs and hip flexors) and extending your extensors (glutes, lats, upper back, hamstrings and calves), I fully recommend you consider doing the opposite:

Flex your extensors and extend your flexors.

In motion, flexor muscles always flex from an extended position and extensor muscles extend from a flexed position. This is how the body learns to work effortlessly and find a balance point between the two.

Adductors adduct from an abducted position and external rotators rotate externally, but from an internally rotated position. Got the picture?

Sit-ups flex your spine towards maximum flexion from a neutral(ish) position, thus encouraging strength in a shortened range whilst not allowing for any extension in the spine and thus limits lengthening in the abdominals.

The only role the abdominals have in motion is to flex the spine from a long, extended position – so please create exercises to do just that and then do the same for all muscles in the body.

Flexing your abs over a Swiss ball is better (more length), BUT anything that lengthens your abs whilst on your feet and incorporates your foot function as well is an awesome way of going about flattening the stomach and opening up the 'eight-pack', baby! Yes, why settle for just six when you can have all eight?

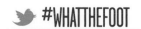

WHAT THE FOOT?

Visualising what the body does in the real world and incorporating it into your exercise and therapy sessions means you are giving the body the tools to do what it does best – seek a way out of pain and get back into peak performance, accessing its hard-wired state of perfection.

What this means for the performance of your feet is that if they do not have the capacity to supinate–pronate–resupinate through centre in the gait cycle then there will not be perfectly optimal movement in the body as a whole.

What there will be is compensatory responses in the ankles, knees, hips, spine, shoulder girdle, shoulders and neck. Ouch!

Naturally, your body will flex up, like a hedgehog, to protect itself from the aggressive external environment we impose upon it each day. This, of course, is purely a perception, for if you teach the body to flow effortlessly and to conserve energy with each step, the brain would relish the opportunity to stand tall and stride out to its full potential, head held high.

When you step outside the comfort zone, there is no option to sink or swim, everybody just swims. If only we all had the guts to overcome our 'fears' and just do it.

NOBODY-EVER-MOVED-ME-ITIS

I could choose many case studies here. The one I have in mind is a lady who met my friend Oliver Dudley (the marathon runner from the first chapter) in a bar, dressed up to the nines – wearing trainers!

The conversation went like this:

"Why are you wearing trainers?"

"Because I can't wear anything else. I have a problem with my feet, which means I can't wear any other footwear, because it hurts so much when I do."

Oliver asked the following question and I think the way he asked it is possibly the reason she called me: "Would you ever entertain the possibility that you could be without pain?" He didn't try to sell a miracle cure, he simply offered her a glimmer of light.

She claimed that of course she would, purely and simply because she wants to get back into her heels! You wouldn't believe how many times I hear that. ☺

She had a condition I have decided to call 'nobody-ever-moved-me-itis'.

The list of treatments she had endured ranged from all manner of physiotherapy and osteopathic remedies to reflexology, acupuncture, MRI scans, X-rays, cortisone injections and more alcohol, please!

Nobody moved her... ever.

It might have been manipulated by physios and osteopaths, but it had never been taught to interact with the ground and reconnect with the rest of the body. Sounds ridiculous doesn't it? To teach a foot to do something it's had no choice but to do all its life?

Well that's what I did. I taught the foot to move, first by re-educating the following patterns:
- Pronation in suspension phase of gait
- Supination in propulsive phase of gait
- Resupination from a pronated position
- Hip extension at appropriate phases
- And incorporated an awareness of spinal extension twice during the gait cycle

WHAT THE FOOT?

Never underestimate the power of the human foot. It brings the five big rules to life and an understanding of it completely transforms the way you think about anatomy and the human body

I did nothing more in those first 30 minutes when she claimed that for the first time in months she was pain free. I hadn't even finished with her yet!

'Nobody-ever-moved-me-itis' is a condition most of you and your clients suffer from. When you are in this position, you are purely subjected to life on the conventional side of the coin like my client was. Yet her solution lay on the other side of the coin, where all unsolvable pain becomes solvable through movement.

Just today I heard about a guy who ruptured his Achilles tendon for the second time in six months. Low-quality rehab and a severe case of 'nobody-ever-moved-me-itis'... the irony is he gave my number to a client with back pain and never called me himself. We'll never know what could have been the outcome.

These two cases are a case in point that, as a practitioner, it is very important to respect the wishes of the patient. Miss Trainers and Mr Achilles both had the opportunity for change in their lives. One took it and the other didn't. She made the choice for a different way and the result was astonishing. He didn't... I hope he still has my number.

Change happens within. At no point ever do I attempt to inflict change on other people – they have to make the choice themselves. The amazing thing about the human body is it responds in this way, too. By introducing new movement patterns and issuing new challenges to the centre of mass within the base of support, the body has the opportunity to change itself. In many other realms of therapy and exercise the trainer or therapist far too often plays the role of 'change agent' and attempts to force

change on the patients. This leads to an ego of 'I did that', which completely takes the emphasis away from the client, which is why I only work with people who have unsolvable physical problems who wish to make that change in their life.

Miss Trainers was running within a week and even more delighted that she could go out in her high heels.

Never underestimate the power of the human foot. It brings the five big rules to life and an understanding of it completely transforms the way you think about anatomy and the human body. To experience change in the foot is one thing, to integrate it into full body movement is another, but to have that change eliminate existing and unsolvable physical problems creates unknown opportunity for you, your clients and your business, too.

All that from the two plates of meat you have dragged around all your life and taken no notice of? Take note: they have been dragging you around and have been managing your performance and functionality since the day you could walk... it's time to show them some gratitude and finally **WAKE THEM UP**, spend some quality time with them and go forth as a perfect partnership...

SUMMARY
YOUR FEET BRING THE FIVE RULES ALIVE

- The foot is perfectly set up to mobilise your mass and generate optimal flow motion.
- The foot is a tripod – timing of contact of the tripod on the ground influences the gait cycle.
- The relationship of the rearfoot and the forefoot is critical.
- Motion at the rearfoot can be described as a type I or a type II motion.
- Big rule #2 – joints ACT, muscles REACT: pronation acts on the muscles of resupination by lengthening them first to activate big rule #1.
- Pronation talks to the hip directly, demanding a response from the big butt muscles.
- Pronation is the trigger for long-term glute activation.
- DO NOT ATTEMPT TO STAMP PRONATION OUT; it is not a terrorist!
- Without pronation you shut down the extensor chain. A dominant flexor chain does not make for a healthy society.
- The foot is designed to adapt to all surfaces (pronation) and react by creating a rigid lever to propel the body forwards (resupination).
- Neutral in the foot is not a solution; experience of the full spectrum in each joint is.
- The foot directly impacts on the centre of mass. If both feet are not identical in posture and movement mechanics, your centre of mass will be influenced and imbalance whips up the kinetic chain.

- No muscles are set up to pronate the foot in motion – gravity does that, leaving the remaining muscles to be considered as resupinators.
- Don't let your patients and clients suffer from 'nobody-ever-moved-me-itis'.

CHAPTER 6:
THE FLOW MOTION MODEL

Each moment the foot is on the floor it is changing shape and using all of its potential characteristics: pronating to adapt to the ground and absorb shock, passing through centre to optimise movement, resupinating and forming a rigid lever to support the toe off and swinging back to complete the cycle

"A man walking is never in balance, but always correcting for imbalance."
Gregory Bateson

One of the implications of understanding the foot is to be able to recognise the impact it has on the gait cycle in human movement.

According to Wikipedia: "Gait is the pattern of movement of the limbs of animals, including humans, and refers to propulsion across a solid substrate by generating reactive forces against it."

Why we use gait as a reference is because it presents a very simple and consistent way of looking at the body in motion. We can assess various moments in the gait cycle where clear whole-body patterns occur.

In terms of timing and observation there is a process the foot takes on the floor and there is a response to this process that occurs elsewhere and everywhere in the body.

Each moment the foot is on the floor it is changing shape and using all of its potential characteristics: pronating to adapt to the ground and absorb shock, passing through centre to optimise movement, resupinating and forming a rigid lever to support the toe off and swinging back to complete the cycle.

Sadly, gait is one of those boring words that not many people care to understand, and gait analysis is something bandied about by podiatrists and shoe shops to sell orthotics and shoes, isn't it? I certainly had followed this approach back in the days of ski boot fitting and selling.

"Whoah, there goes another over-pronating foot! You'll need an orthotic, a new ski boot/trainer and a new pair of socks while you are at it. Why not?" I still see this shotgun approach today, hearing tell of the owner of a well-known spa in the UK describing selling 'gait analysis' and 'off-the-shelf orthotics' that accompany the assessment as akin to shooting fish in a barrel. Spa = fat people = flat feet = an extra £270 out of each person we can get to walk over the footplate...!

This is not how gait analysis should be perceived. Little did I know when I ventured down the human movement track that gait analysis was actually a highly organised way of observing optimal and suboptimal patterns in the body and, beyond assessment, to actually optimise gait through movement would have huge carry over to the wellbeing of the person.

Mostly, gait is used in the following areas:
- General assessment of a person
- Shoe fitting (in particular running)
- Podiatry – observing the lower limbs

WHAT THE FOOT?

It can be used in an incredibly powerful way when you use it not just to determine what the body is doing, i.e. limping, but to determine exactly how it's doing what it's doing and how what it is doing differs from what it should or could be doing in a more efficient manner.

One of the things I have always professed is that I only discuss what the body actually does as opposed to what we think it does. It's so often the case that a student informs me of what he thinks his body is doing, thanks to the anatomical brainwashing he has had in school/university or on a training course, and then when I ask him to describe what it is doing, it's often different and shows up as a surprise to that particular student.

"Dur," being the appropriate response. My other favourite student response is "It's the 'bleedin' obvious!" and you can see Sean describe that feeling on this video link: **www.whatthefoot.co.uk/ bleedinobvious**

Anatomy is difficult to understand and the modern way of learning it, in an attempt to simplify it, has taken us way off course with what is really going on – actually overcomplicating things, if that's possible. Gait, however, shines a light on human movement in a way I could never have imagined and by studying it, slowing it down and working with it – not just the lower limbs, but the whole body – has given new wings to the understanding and delivery of educating human movement.

Flow motion

The model of gait that is taught at AiM is what I call the 'flow motion model'. It is the study of what appears to really happen when efficient and flowing gait is observed and has been deduced through the use of slow motion – slowing the body down to get a clear picture of what is happening in each major structure and each joint in the three dimensions of human movement from the foot and journeying upwards through the kinetic chain. For a quick reminder, if necessary, check back to the three dimensions portrayed on pages 32 and 33.

For me, the flow motion model is a revised model of gait, which embraces movement of the whole body and not just the foot alone.

Walking is something we are destined to do from birth; it's imprinted in our DNA. It defines us as human. In human gait, there is a noticeable pattern that we leave behind on a force plate that is called our 'centre of pressure'. This pattern becomes predictable and informative. The model of flow motion is based on five phases along this pathway of mean pressure under the foot, with each phase interconnecting up the whole body. We can see from this model that the way we walk affects everything from our physiology to how well we carry out our daily and sporting activities. All movement from walking and running to more diverse sports such as skiing, tennis and field sports can be mapped to the flow motion model.

There are countless running coaches, but few walking coaches. Well, I have some news for you:

If you can't walk, you can't run.

When problems arise in running, it's normal to look at a person's running technique with little consideration for how they walk. There will very clearly be a problem with the way the person walks; noticeably, we see the

I only discuss what the body actually does as opposed to what we think it does

→ OVERLAPPED IMAGE OF OPTIMAL GAIT AND INHIBITED GAIT. SHOULD THERE BE A HIP HIKE OR NOT? THE FLOW MOTION MODEL WILL TELL YOU AND, AS GAIT SPECIALISTS, YOU LOOK FOR WHAT THE BODY CANNOT DO OR DOES NOT DO WELL

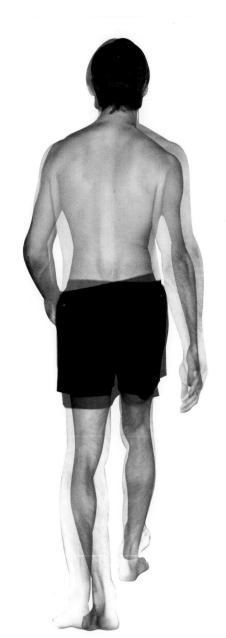

same inhibitions in walking gait translate to running gait. It's easier to observe and, using the flow motion model, easier to treat.

The flow motion model teaches people to walk better, more fluidly, with enhanced posture. It enables people to appreciate full motion at all joints in the body and thus experience improved range and tone in all muscles. Once we get that right, running becomes a breeze. The carry over is immediate. Better running is a natural consequence of improving walking gait. In fact, if you swap run in that sentence for any other sporting activity – ski, football, dance – none of which come easy if walking is hard – you can begin to see the power of the flow motion model. If I'm right, then it certainly pays to understand walking better as it will give you the keys to understand a person's running inhibitions.

SO WHAT DOES THE FLOW MOTION MODEL GIVE ME?

Imagine for the heel to touch the ground there was an optimal way of it doing so and for that to happen a series of interconnected events must happen, too: the hip must do something special, the spine something extraordinary, with one arm opposing the action of the other arm... and... and... and, you'd be interested in the information you could get from that wouldn't you? What if the same phenomenon happened in each moment that the foot is in contact with the ground? What if each moment dictated a wholesale change in the joint alignment of the whole skeleton? Would that be groundbreaking? I'd certainly be interested and I can tell you for nothing, that this is exactly what is going on.

Working with movement can be simplified as simply taking the human body, watching it walk and plotting the movement of the whole body in gait, matching it up with the flow motion model and looking for the difference between optimal and suboptimal gait; in other words, looking for aspects of the flow motion model that are not happening when they should. The clues lie in this process – the process of determining dynamic anatomical posture coupled with static skeletal posture.

The inhibited gait that you are observing in the client should be viewed as a persistent habit that the client is displaying. It represents the only way the person knows how to walk and highlights the most energy-conserving state that the client can currently access (either because of any pain or in avoidance of a pain, for example). This becomes their functional gait, the one the brain adds most value to, and makes getting from A to B possible for the client.

I have scanned clients in static stance who stand with 72% weight through their right foot and upwards of 50% bodyweight standing through their right heel. I have scanned these people two weeks apart, without treatment, and the numbers don't change. It's a habit, an efficient way of standing, despite their performance level sliding way down the bell curve.

It's the same for gait: two weeks apart and the patterns displayed in gait don't change, favouring one leg over the other and highlighting forefoot and rearfoot imbalances along the way.

The way you walk is a habit that is unchanging. It's a pattern that you replay again and again, step after step. What's important to take from this is that faulty gait is a way of being for the client – it doesn't get better one day and worse the next; it's consistent, persistent and limiting in every way.

The slightest attempt to change this pattern to access its hard-wired state will have a far greater impact than massaging the sore muscles, foam rolling the soft tissue and prescribing a stretching protocol. Inhibited gait, via the five rules, will always return an effective treatment back to a state of discomfort if the gait is not challenged and introduced to centre. When I finally got round to treating these people: the scan results changed instantly. As soon as the clients' dynamic and static stance postures were restored back to the optimal patterns dictated by the flow motion model, their discomfort would simply drop away, moving them from pain towards performance.

The response in the body, displayed by the digitised scans, is simple and clear for all to see. The body simply moves back towards centre.

I want you to stand up and place 70% of your bodyweight through your right foot, and then the majority of your weight through your right heel, maintaining contact through both forefeet and the left heel as well. How does that feel? Comfortable? Imagine walking around on that for the past eight years?

What if nobody ever offered you the chance to change it and you remained oblivious of that possibility for years? Given a choice of a better stance position and a more efficient gait cycle, you'd choose it, wouldn't you?

This happens every time – the body recognises new efficient ways of movement and instantly accesses them to reduce the pain in the body and pressure on certain joints... and it moves back towards the centre.

The way you walk is a habit that is unchanging. It's a pattern that you replay again and again, step after step. What's important to take from this is that faulty gait is a way of being for the client – it doesn't get better one day and worse the next; it's consistent, persistent and limiting in every way

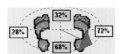

↑ BEFORE

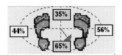

↑ AFTER

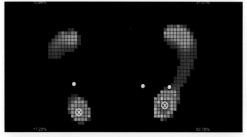

↑ BEFORE ↓ AFTER

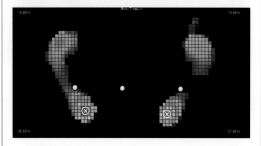

In the top image you can see the dot representing the centre of mass shifting back towards the centre, having reduced the amount of pressure placed through the right heel from 50% to 39% — not out of the woods yet, but already the pain is greatly reduced.

In the image above you can see the shift in the same client's bodyweight over the same time period as the client moves from 72% bodyweight through the right side down to 56% — almost reverting to ideal, which would be 50%.

This case study has already been represented on page 106, in the section entitled 'Hardwired'.

At this point, the whole skeleton changes: each joint in the body changes position and any compressive forces, torsional forces or sheering forces in the joint system change, too.

Each joint finds centre, the muscle system adapts instantaneously to manage the new skeletal framework and everything gets easier. More importantly, a significant amount of pain drops away. Gone!

PATTERNS

So you are probably wondering what these patterns are?

It is an established concept that the body travels through a variety of phases in the gait cycle.
- In each phase the foot is in a different position to the previous phase.
- At each phase the joint system of the whole body is in a different position to the previous phase — from head to toe.
- This ultimately means that the muscle system, too, is in a different position to the previous phase.

These phases are commonly known as:
- heel strike
- foot flat
- mid-stance
- early toe off
- late toe off
- swing phase (early)
- swing phase (late)

What is not commonly known and discussed is the position of the whole body in each of the phases and the impact on the whole body when it is not moving efficiently through these phases.

- How does the body adapt when a flat foot moves through these phases? How does the body adapt when a supinated high-arched foot moves through these phases?

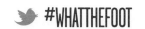

WHAT THE FOOT?

● How does the body adapt when the two feet react differently to each other through the phases?

Have you considered that the way the heel hits the ground directly impacts the effort required to travel through the phases efficiently? If the heel strike is suboptimal, the subsequent phases will be purely compensatory. In this case the body will firstly try to get back on track with the model of flow motion and secondly give up so as to concentrate on getting the other foot on the ground and keep momentum going forwards.

This compensatory pattern is repeated again and again and becomes the habit by which it masters the task of gait. Only somebody who understands whole-body motion in gait, the five big rules of human movement, the intricacies of foot function in these phases and the three-dimensional approach to restoring any missing patterns in the gait cycle can have a major and instant impact on these compensations.

It is these six movement patterns that have put many an athlete back on track, footballers back on the pitch and a smile on the face of the hundreds of 'in pain' and 'underperforming' individuals that have come my way and, indeed, the way of AiM students and graduates.

PHASES

When we look at a dynamic pressure plate scan on a force plate, we are presented with a pattern, determined by average and peak pressures, that the foot has taken throughout its contact with the ground and from this we can determine whole-body patterns that occur simultaneously.

Similar to static stance, it's as if it's possible to appreciate a hologram of the person's body rising above the image on the screen and all kinds of things stand out: from overstretched adductors to shortened hip flexors as well as dominance and inhibition in spinal movement.

The phases of gait in the flow motion model are relative to the pathway taken by the centre of pressure through the foot in dynamic gait, as in the images to the right.

Most feet don't look like this when you first scan them. Most people I work with have pain. When the scan begins to follow this white curve it is synonymous with one thing: the person has begun to move effortlessly and without pain. So what is it?

The white line is the centre of pressure. The centre of pressure is representative of the centre of gravity as it moves through the foot. The relationship between the centre of pressure, centre of gravity and centre of mass is very special indeed.

We have already seen how the centre of gravity is represented on the floor directly and vertically beneath the centre of mass, and the centre of gravity becomes the centre of pressure when it is under the foot and pressure and forces are exerted about this point.

It has been described as a dance between the centres of pressure and gravity, never quite together, but never too far apart. My best guess is they would follow a wave-like pattern in relation to each other.

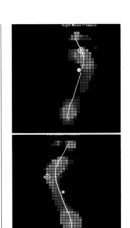

↑ **OPTIMISED CENTRE OF PRESSURE PATHWAYS FOR SMOOTH FLOW MOTION**

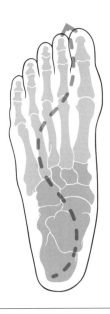

WHAT THE FOOT?

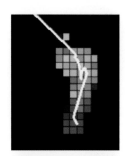

⬆ FLOW MOTION: PRESENT
FROM OUR EARLIEST DAYS

That said, the two are so close that, for simplicity's sake, I assume and teach they are both one and the same thing and it makes for an easier explanation.

Ultimately, take away from this that the centres of mass, gravity and pressure form a vertical line from lumbar spine to the floor through the foot as we walk. Taking this into account, and by following the white line, we can see how the centre of mass, aka L4/L5, passes along the foot, hovering directly over the centre of pressure.

The talus, too, in the transverse plane follows this white line perfectly, as does the knee, which sits directly above the talus bone, inseparable in its motion.*

Do I need to bring up the knee over toe debacle again? The knee follows that little white line with every step you take and is never static in one position, travelling, ideally, either side of that 2nd toe midline.

So we can tell a lot from simply looking at this line and its shape. If it doesn't look like the 's' curve we see in the gait image (right) then we know that the flow of movement can be improved and may well be indicative of a person's pain.

Top left is a closer image of my 14-month-old daughter's gait pathway, which I showed earlier in the book. Can you see the line of flow motion present? I realise I'm cherry-picking here to some extent, but I also see it's a pretty close fit and does reveal that the centre of pressure for optimal motion is present from our earliest days.

SIX PHASES OF HUMAN MOVEMENT

Interestingly, gait is nothing more than a forward projection of our centre of mass. As our centre of mass moves along the little white line known as the centre of pressure we can watch the foot pass through the phases of gait. Mapping out what the body does over each phase of gait creates the understanding of whole-body motion relative to the foot in motion.

THE FLOW MOTION MODEL

At each point where there is a significant change in the position of the joint system, we can highlight a point and call it a phase. As a result of this process – pretty much a whole summer of me moving to and fro over a space of about 5mm trying to be clear about what exactly is going on in each space! – six phases of human movement were born.

They are:
- strike phase
- suspension (load) phase
- transition phase
- shift phase
- propulsion phase
- swing phase

Each phase impacts the centre of mass in such a way that skeletal alignment changes and impacts on muscle tissue, which is perfectly set up to defend the movement so it does not stray too far from where it needs to be to maximise efficiency and minimise effort in the cycle.

When the centre of pressure passes through the foot optimally, a state of flow is experienced in the

*Note: this is only true of the talus and the knee up until the curve returns back from the little toe area, back towards the big toe in the later phases of this foot's gait cycle – we call it 'shift phase': more on this later.

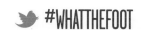

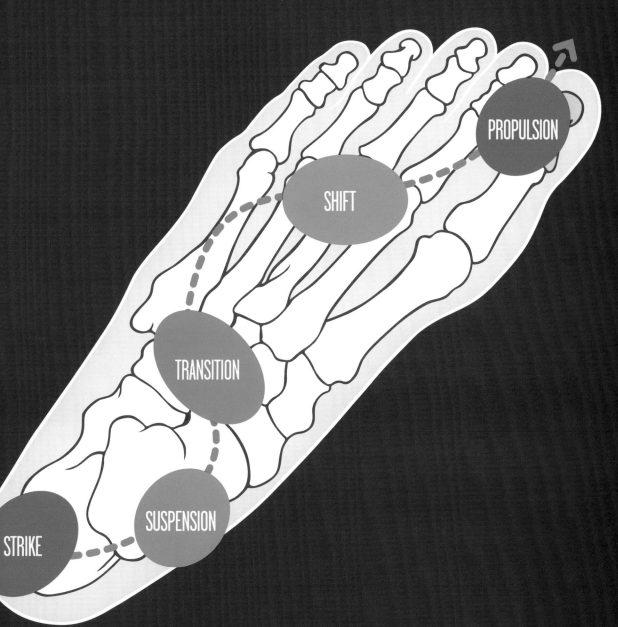

WHAT THE FOOT?

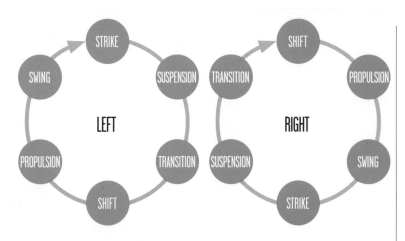

body, where balance is attained and your gait or walk to work becomes effortless.

TIMINGS

Unsurprisingly, gait is a two-legged action, so whilst one foot is passing through its relevant phase, the opposite must be passing through a different phase.

Reading across the circles above, we can see the following phases occur simultaneously:

- The strike phase (left) and the shift phase (right) occur together.
- The suspension phase and the propulsion phase occur together.
- The transition phase and the swing phase occur together.

Effectively then, there are three moments to look for in a person's gait to get a clear and objective viewpoint on what is happening in that person's body. What muscles they aren't using very well and what joints are being over or underutilised... and all too often it becomes very clear as to why a massage, or localised treatment on the site of

pain, has had little or no effect when the way they walk compromises the area of pain with each step they take.

Picture a faulty gait pattern leading to hip pain and now visualise a couch-based treatment that focuses on the hip and surrounding tissue. Post session, once the patient returns to their habitual pattern of gait, the hip problem slowly resurfaces as the client walks out the door, only to be back soon for another dose of the same. This is not the failing of the practitioner, it's the failing of the anatomical model at large — the result of focusing on only one side of the coin.

These three phases make it a lot simpler to learn and 'see' when working with a client.

Once you have seen which gait phase isn't working, or the repetitive patterns that the client is continuously using, it's a very simple approach of using the exercise or movement pattern that corresponds to each phase of the flow motion model.

FAULTY GAIT PATTERNS AND STRUCTURAL ANOMALIES

The interesting thing about the joint actions experienced through each of these phases is that there is not a single joint action available to the body that does not occur during these five phases of the flow motion model.

For example, a varus forefoot is what is ordinarily described as a pathology or a 'dysfunction'. Despite that, a varus forefoot — noticeably recognised by a forefoot inversion/supination — is a necessary joint motion for optimal gait to occur and occurs in one of the phases. A valgus forefoot is equally expected to be present somewhere in the gait cycle. So are we actually noticing 'dysfunctions' and pathologies, or are we simply noticing people stuck in relative gait phases that they can't get out of? That is definitely #footforthought.

If every three-dimensional joint motion that we have available to us happens somewhere in the gait cycle, then does it not stand to reason that we should be seeking to access each of these movements? How to get into them and how to get out of them?

Have you seen a patient stuck in right thoracic rotation?
That happens in the gait cycle.

Have you seen a patient stuck in anterior tilt?
That happens in the gait cycle.

Have you seen a patient with a scoliosis?
That happens in the gait cycle.

What about an occipital bone (base of skull) that is raised on one side and rotated to the other?
That also happens in the gait cycle.

Most likely, what is not happening is that the structure is not being given the opportunity to move from one position into another in conjunction with the rest of the whole body. It gets stuck and that naturally influences the gait cycle.

CHICKEN OR EGG?
Does the perceived anomaly change gait or did the person's gait cause the anomaly?

Most likely, any change is a global consequence of how we adapt our structure to the way we function as a result of a slide down the bell curves mentioned earlier in the book. A structural change in the body will change the gait cycle and a small change in the gait cycle will reach up to alter the overall structure of the body, especially when the change is made in an integrated environment. Let's not look past the point, though, that the structural anomalies you are witnessing in your assessments actually form a vital and necessary part of the gait cycle and should be encouraged and mobilised as opposed to shut down and minimised. You will never find a joint motion in the body that does not occur in my flow motion model.

What might be useful is to look for the moments where these phases happen and you can begin to look at the shapes the human form takes during gait.

RULES OF FLOW MOTION PHASES
In order to determine what each of these phases looks like, I defined a set of rules to help us recognise the foot posture relative to each phase:
- Strike phase – heel on ground, toes off
- Suspension phase – tripod on ground pronating
- Transition phase – tripod on ground supinating
- Shift phase – heel off ground, toes on, supinating (stage I)
- Propulsion phase - heel off ground, toes on, supinating (stage II)
- Swing phase – zero point of contact with the ground

These rules give us a start point to both witness motion through the phases and to begin to work our way up the kinetic chain to figure out the whole-body posture in relation to each phase.

WHAT THE FOOT?

The overriding parameter in human movement, static stance and gait is the brain's perception of what is optimal for you

It also emerges that once we have an awareness of the position of the whole-body posture, then it becomes clear as to which muscles actually play a key role in decelerating the skeletal posture for each phase.

DOMINANT LOADING MUSCLES (RESPONSIBLE FOR DECELERATION)

- Strike phase – hamstrings, FHL, lumbar erectors
- Suspension phase – gluteals, VMO, hamstrings, resupinators
- Transition phase – cross abdominals, peroneals, hamstrings
- Shift phase – adductors, rhomboids
- Propulsion phase – hip flexors, abdominals

SIX EXERCISES THAT CHANGE YOUR WORLD

Six phases means six movement patterns or six exercises. That means six movements that follow the five big rules and dramatically change the way the brain perceives the role of its own human body.

Introducing efficient patterns of movement to the brain is a rapid and reliable approach to upgrading whole-body function.

This approach changes the client's world as it opens up an incredible amount of opportunity and alleviates any risk of exposure to emergency situations, where the body could be at risk of injury. There is an anatomical shift that takes place in the person, never to return again.

In six years, I have never seen a client return back to the physical posture they carried at the time of their first session. It simply doesn't happen. The overriding parameter in human movement, static stance and

gait is the brain's perception of what is optimal for the body in terms of:

- efficiency
- energy conservation
- effort
- ▶ Yes, it is harder to stand wonky than straight!
- ▶ Yes, it is harder to walk with a limp than without!
- ▶ Yes, it's way more effort to run when both feet work differently to each other!

Oh, and, yes, you are more likely to get injured or experience pain or limitations in performance in any of the above scenarios pre rebalancing the whole physical system and transforming the brain's perception of your physical you.

Six simple exercises and you'll press the big reset button on the body and be ready to go again, free, liberated and with a sense of opportunity about you.

DISCLAIMER

I am choosing not to give you the movements per se in this book, primarily because it would take too long to cross all the barriers of usage, timings of each joint motion and muscular interaction at each phase. Not to mention the fact that I am unwilling to expose your clients at this point to any risk because, with all due respect, you don't yet know and understand the 'ins' and 'outs' of working with the body in this way – it takes students a few days to get comfortable with the concept and, while they can get great results in just a few days, it takes a while to become competent and confident with the system.

My motivation is your results and the results of your clients. My mission is to change the way we think about pain in our bodies from it being a burden to a mere pattern breakdown or alteration that simply needs rewiring.

My mission will be based purely on its success and, at this stage, sending out the tools for use is not the sensible way forward. My intention for you in this book is to grasp the value of working with movement and seek to learn more and more about it.

It is, quite simply, the most powerful tool I have worked with for the human body. Coupled with an excellent physio, osteopath or chiropractor, you can cover all angles in managing a person's physical discomfort. What would be even better, is if you are already an excellent physio, chiropractor or osteopath and had the tool of movement under your belt. It's safe to say you would be a force to be reckoned with!

FASCIA IN MOTION

I want to mention briefly the role of fascia in the moving body. Fascia, in particular since the release of Tom Myers' book, has taken on a huge role in the fitness and therapy industry especially. I would always recommend getting hold of his book, *Anatomy Trains*, to see and experience the fascial lines he has developed as a way of understanding the interconnectedness of the soft and hard tissue in the human body.

Fascia envelops everything, from each bone and muscle fibre to each nerve and organ in the body. Tom goes as far as to say that "the muscle is dead" and all that we are is a mass of soft tissue surrounding a skeleton – forgive me if that statement is not 100% accurate. In which case it makes complete sense to map the fascia over the body and take a good look at its role in human motion.

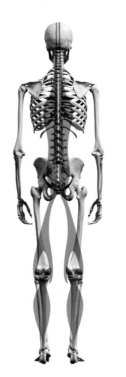
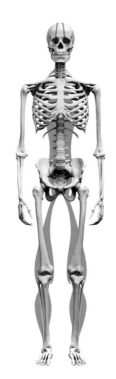
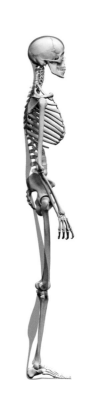

↑ SAGITTAL PLANE LINE: SUPERFICIAL BACK LINE (AFTER MYERS)

THREE DIMENSIONAL

The fascial lines outlined in Anatomy Trains are naturally three dimensional in nature. Separated down to each plane, there exist the following lines of fascia:

- Sagittal plane – superficial front and back line
- Frontal plane – lateral line and deep front line
- Transverse plane – spiral line and the front and back functional lines

Looking at both static and dynamic stance, it's possible to witness the role that whole lines of fascia play in managing the mass of the human body... and it is simply beautiful.

WHAT THE FOOT?

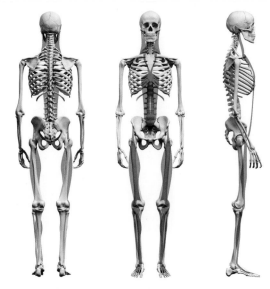

↑ SAGITTAL PLANE LINE: SUPERFICIAL FRONT LINE (AFTER MYERS)

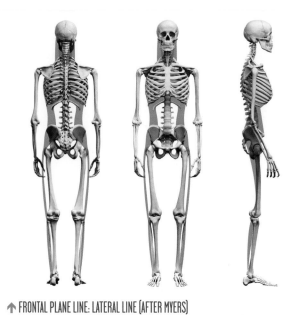

↑ FRONTAL PLANE LINE: LATERAL LINE (AFTER MYERS)

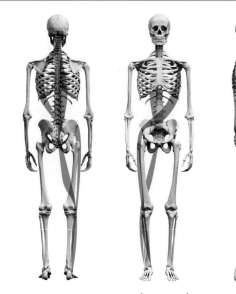

↑ FRONTAL PLANE LINE: DEEP FRONT LINE (AFTER MYERS)

↑ TRANSVERSE PLANE LINE: SPIRAL LINE (AFTER MYERS)

STATIC STANCE

As we have discussed before, static stance is successful providing the centre of gravity does not pass beyond the base of support, and is optimal the closer it is to centre within that base of support.

Since each line of fascia runs from head to toe (barring the front and back functional lines, which are made up of the powerhouse muscles of lats, glutes, obliques and hip flexors), it stands to reason that any movement in the foot or head will change the length tensions in the fascial lines.

Back to our base of support and centre of gravity discussion, we mentioned earlier that the centre of gravity is never still and, from centre, would proceed outwards towards the boundaries of the base of support. If we change the word 'muscle' in big rule #1 and #2 to 'fascia' then nothing really changes here. As the centre of gravity challenges the base of support, it indicates that the skeleton is moving away from centre and thus there is a tension exchange in the whole fascial system. The fascial line is lengthening and must react to bring the body back to its centre and optimal restful position.

Visualise one of those trampolines with a net standing up around it to prevent the kids from falling off. That's the fascia preventing the body's centre of mass from leaving its own base of support!

FLOW MOTION

Dynamically we see the same thing happening. The muscles that are being asked to perform their role at each phase of the cycle correspond nicely to the lines of fascia drawn up by Mr Myers. The lines react

to control skeletal movement and optimise it at the same time by executing perfectly timed reactions to get the body fluidly from one phase to the other.

Interestingly enough, the gait cycle can be broken down into planar dominance at each phase:
- Strike phase – sagittal plane dominant
- Suspension phase – frontal plane dominant
- Transition phase – transverse plane dominant
- Shift phase – frontal plane dominant
- Propulsion phase – sagittal plane dominant
- Swing phase – transverse plane dominant

However, since each of these phases corresponds with another simultaneously, there is never a single line of fascia that is active at one time.

As we said before:
- The strike phase (left) and the shift phase (right) occur together
- The suspension phase and the propulsion phase occur together
- The transition phase and the swing phase occur together

So:
- The left side superficial back line and right side deep front line load up together
- The left side lateral line and right side superficial front line load up together
- The left side spiral line and the right side spiral line load up together

For example, if the left leg is in the suspension phase, and the right leg is in the propulsion phase, then the frontal fascial lateral line is active along with the sagittally orientated superficial front line. The fact that the one leg forward and one leg back factor

Visualise one of those trampolines with a net standing up around it to prevent the kids from falling off. That's the fascia preventing the body's centre of mass from leaving its own base of support!

WHAT THE FOOT?

LEFT SIDE

- STRIKE SUPERFICIAL BACK LINE
- SWING SPIRAL LINE
- SUSPENSION LATERAL LINE
- PROPULSION SUPERFICIAL FRONT LINE
- TRANSITION SPIRAL LINE
- SHIFT DEEP FRONT LINE

RIGHT SIDE

- SHIFT DEEP FRONT LINE
- TRANSITION SPIRAL LINE
- PROPULSION SUPERFICIAL FRONT LINE
- SUSPENSION LATERAL LINE
- SWING SPIRAL LINE
- STRIKE SUPERFICIAL BACK LINE

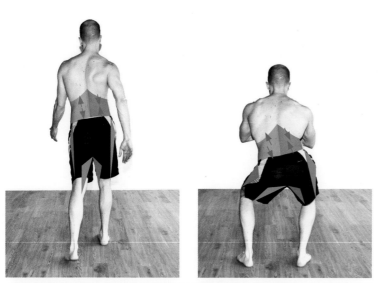

↑WHEN THE PELVIS TRAVELS TO THE RIGHT IN EITHER A SQUAT OR IN GAIT YOU CAN SEE THE ADAPTATION IN THE FASCIAL LINES, SHORTENING AND LENGTHENING IN REACTION TO THE SKELETAL POSITION

creates a rotation in the pelvis and thus impacts on the cross-functional lines in the transverse plane, is sufficient to highlight that there is actually no separation in the fascia of the whole body during gait. Since the whole body is moving, the whole fascial system must adapt to that movement to generate perfect function. The fascial system is yet another whole-body entity and we can neither ignore it nor break it down to understand the value of it in terms of movement, posture, wellbeing and performance.

When it breaks down we simply see adaptation in the fascial lines on one side compared to the other. If, for example, the pelvis travels laterally further to the right than the left in gait or, indeed, even in a squat, then we would notice the lateral line about the pelvis on the right-hand side lengthening, with the lateral line about the pelvis on the left-hand side shortening. There will be a corresponding adaptation

🐦 #WHATTHEFOOT

WHAT THE FOOT?

in the deep front line as well, with the left deep front (in particular adductor) lengthening and the opposite shortening, and a habit being created about this moment. Think left groin pain, right TFL/ITB pain for a basic example.

What if we, in this case, could create a simple movement that enabled this person to do the opposite pattern, in an upright position – and in a pain-free environment? To get them to experience more lateral shift to the left to rebalance? Would we be informing the brain of opposing length tensions so it can rediscover its optimal alignment – the one it's hardwired to find and subconsciously knows exactly where it is? I think so.

ZERO TENSION

Fascia is perhaps best observed in movement as a tension exchange as opposed to a lengthening or shortening. Notice I don't really separate the notion of muscle and fascia – and, actually, it serves you to recognise that muscle enveloped in the fascia is best observed as a tension exchange as well.

Lengthening whole fascial lines in a single 'stretch' is more like yoga than movement. Absolutely nothing wrong with that, except for the fact that walking and movement defined by keeping the head over the feet looks very little like yoga! (Personal note: I love yoga so I'm not bashing it here.)

Walking is a tensional exchange whereby each step sees aspects of a fascial line lengthen while other parts of it shorten. For instance, the superficial front line crosses the pelvis via the quads and the rectus abdominus – arguably, the hip flexors could be included here, too. When the foot is in contact with the ground in suspension phase, the hip is flexed and

the spine is extended, thus aspects of the front line are short below the hip and long above it.

Tension is created in the soft tissue when it lengthens: ordinarily, tension is defined when two things move apart. Tension is opposed by compression. Away from centre, there will be elements of both tension and compression in the physical system – this leads to a natural slide down the bell curve and a downgrade in performance or increase in possibility of pain or risk of injury.

If we assume that in centre the skeleton is neutralised, and the muscles and fascial lines are at resting length, then we can assume that there is little or no tension in the fascial system as a whole.

We call this 'zero tension'. It's not strictly zero since there is always an element of movement and vibration in the system due to the fact we cannot stand still, but at least in optimal stance this minimal amount of tension is equalised throughout the system, i.e. it is in balance, and this is a more accurate explanation of the term 'zero tension'.

"Zero tension is when tension is evenly distributed and equalised throughout the system as a whole."

TENSION ALGEBRA

In a perfectly 100% functioning human body there must always be balance – much like in a mathematical equation. In algebra, for instance, if we remove something from one side of the equation, we must add it to the other to equate balance.

It's no different in the human body and fascial or muscle system. Remember how some muscles can be long in two dimensions and short in one or vice

Zero tension is when tension is evenly distributed and equalised throughout the system as a whole

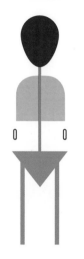

0   0

↑ ZERO TENSION = TENSION
BALANCED ON BOTH SIDES

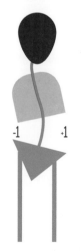

-1   +1

↑ TENSION INCREASED ON
RIGHT, REDUCED ON LEFT AND
TENSION IS EQUATED TO ZERO
(-1 -1 = 0)

versa? It's merely how the body is equating tension throughout the system to manage the mass and generate optimal movement for any given skeletal position. Refer back to the three cups explanation on page 100.

Let's look at a lateral flexion:
A) In neutral spine or centre, tension is balanced on both sides (a = b)

B) In the left laterally flexed spine, tension is increased on the right (+1) and removed from the left (–1) ➜ a–1 = b+1

Tension is equated yet we can perceive it as imbalanced. Here's a painful scenario:
C) The left lateral flexion has increased tension on the right (+5) but this time tension has been transferred through the whole body to equate balance and we see areas of compression to the value of –1 in five other areas of the body. Either way, we see something like this to equate the balance.

a+5 = b1.c1.d1.e1.f1

In all three scenarios, balance is maintained, A) is pain free, B) could be pain free within normal parameters and C) is a problem for the body. At no point have we physically added or taken away from its 100% functionality, but the slider of perceived function is lowered the greater the tensional exchange.

I imagine that went over most people's heads. It would mine if I wasn't actually writing it. I hope to summarise the point by saying that balance is equal to there being minimal tension in the system, and

pain and inhibition is always present where there is evidence of increased compression and tension in the system.

In movement, we are never ever in centre, always moving away from it, towards and hopefully through it, and always operating in three inseparable dimensions. This means that all muscles, all fascia, all organs, all joints and the whole nervous system are never ever stable and never ever isolated.

Whilst you might be thinking that everything goes completely against the grain here, and you'd be right, I hope I can bring it alive for you in the next section.

I do not see evidence of a stable, mobile, stable pattern in the skeletal system. I only see consistent and perpetual movement occurring at each stage in the gait cycle and in all manners of movement. Pelvic, lumbar and thoracic structures all moving simultaneously (some to a lesser degree than others, yet moving all the same) and when they don't, it equates to problems. It is fair to say that there are structures that are more stable than others, but those 'stable' structures, in reality, are never ever stable.

These problems always show up in the flow motion model. Once fully understood, the flow motion model makes it easy for us to assess how our patients walk, the movements they favour and the movements they omit. More often than not, these patterns point the finger to why your patient is experiencing pain in that particular place, and built into the model is also a solution–based process that will guide your patient to find centre following the five big rules to get them out of pain and back to peak performance.

WHAT THE FOOT?

CASE STUDY

AiM and Kinesis Myofascial Integration (KMI) Structural Integration

"Sometime during level three, the full implications for what AiM means for anyone doing bodywork hit me, and the way we should observe the human body was changed forever. The blindfolds were off, and all of my prior knowledge fitted perfectly with this new concept. AiM is systemic – it connects the dots of our fragmented view of the body in a meaningful, coherent way. Understanding AiM's philosophy and the flow motion model/gait cycle and what it entails should be of primary importance for anyone interested in the human body. When you understand this work, it feels like basic knowledge you couldn't possibly be without. KMI also works on a systemic level, which is why the combination of AiM and KMI is so interesting and opens up a whole new domain. Seeing and recognising patterns in the body can be understood on a higher level of complexity; things can seem more complex, but also appear simpler, because to look at the body in this way makes sense and it can be seen from a more coherent perspective. We can appreciate more what it means to be a fully developed kinesthetic human being.

Above all it is a game changer for practitioners and the potential you can achieve with your clients and with yourself. My work has shifted into one big creative experiment. I would recommend to anyone doing bodywork or Structural Integration, to come and join me in this greater vista." **Martin Lundgren, KMI and AiM practitioner,** Halmstad, Sweden

SUMMARY

- The flow motion model is a description of what the whole body does in gait.
- It changes gait analysis from an assessment tool to a corrective tool.
- Walking gait is a habit. It's repetitive, step after step, and is unchanging unless intervention occurs. Global intervention using the flow motion model gives the body and brain the movements back that they have been unable to use.
- The centre of pressure is the journey your mass takes through the gait cycle. Deviations in its pathway highlight flaws in the system as a whole.
- When we see what's missing and add it back using movement, the system changes and manages its mass differently.
- Since one foot passes through one phase while the other foot passes through another, we shift from six phases to three global movements.
- Every single possible structural anomaly shows up in the gait cycle somewhere.
- The fascial system maps perfectly onto the flow motion model, connecting fascial lines to key phases in the model.
- All movement away from centre generates tension and compression relationships. The goal is zero tension – imbalance will always lead to increased tension and increased compression.

"AiM is systemic – it connects the dots of our fragmented view of the body in a meaningful, coherent way."

BIBLIOGRAPHY

MYERS T, 2001, 2009, 2013
ANATOMY TRAINS, EDINBURGH:
ELSEVIER

CHAPTER 7: CORE MOBILITY (THE SPINE IN MOTION)

"Everything is in motion. Everything flows. Everything is vibrating." William Hazlitt (1778-1830)

As an outcome of studying human movement, there are several reasons why I have come to the conclusion that to stabilise the core is not a sole solution.

- Nothing is stable in the body from the ground up, with the feet in a constant state of motion or dynamic equilibrium.
- Our centre of mass, located at L4/L5, is in a persistent state of movement.
- When something does not move, it hurts or its potential is enormously limited.
- All movement is an experience of a three-dimensional spectrum or continuum – a single point on this spectrum cannot be portrayed as movement!
- The body benefits hugely by challenging its base of support and movement is necessary to do this.

Movement and stance thus can be described as below:
The circle and the dot: mobility inside, stability outside.

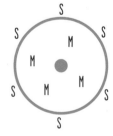

It does not take a three-year PhD to grasp this, by the way; purely a foot scan and a group of students in a room. Remember the star chart diagram on page 68. It should help you appreciate two things: 1) we are never stable; and 2) the eccentric – isometric – concentric patterns of movement.

Here I define it diagrammatically as the circle – which defines our experience of possible movement – and the dot – which defines our awareness of centre; the dot representing your centre of mass and the circle being the perimeter of your base of support, or put another way, the maximal appreciation in the somatosensory cortex of the brain of what motion is actually possible around a specific point (in this case, neutral).

A quick reminder is that once the centre of mass leaves the base of support, we must alter our stance or fall over. The less movement we experience inside our base of support means our perception of that base will be smaller and the risk of falling over or need for compensation to optimise movement will be greater.

If the dot represents your centre point and the circle represents the perimeter of your base of support, then what we notice is that mobility is always present inside the circle.

As we approach the perimeter of the circle we approach the isometric moment of muscular contraction, which lies in between the eccentric and concentric muscular contractions. Thus stability (or

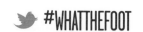

stillness) actually takes place at the outer edge of the circle, YET as an industry, currently, our intention is to build stability around the dot (neutral) inside the circle.

Focusing on stability is akin to there being no awareness of the circle. This in turn means that we can have no understanding of possible ranges or, worse, possibilities in movement potential. You are stuck in the comfort zone that I described earlier, feeling strong and stable, but unable to fully explore your movement potential. You might be thinking that you do heavily work on stabilising your core or the core muscles of your clients; you only need to look at the number of athletes who this approach fails and the number of injuries that continually return from their dormant existence, to have some basic understanding that this concept might largely be flawed.

In actual fact, core stability is not a bad thing to do, providing we then integrate the work throughout the whole body. Core stabilisation is just one part of a solution we have available for our clients. Once again, I'm wondering why the world at large is not focusing on BOTH mobilisation and stabilisation of the core.

STABILITY THROUGH MOBILITY?

To stabilise your body around neutral, and in particular your core, limits movement in the spine whilst also limiting the experience and size of the circle, which represents full movement potential.

All that your core muscles and brain become aware of is the dot without the circle...

What am I in the centre of?

In the model of stability we teach the body to neutralise and stabilise about this point... but how on earth is your body supposed to know where the actual centre is, when you have no idea what you are supposed to be in the centre of?

How can we know where centre is if we don't know where the boundary or limits to our centre are?

You need to experience the border of your potential to even get close to finding your optimal centre point. This is done using movement – full, integrated human movement – accessing all possible ranges, broken down into movement patterns, that the body freely accesses every step of every day. Stabilising inside the circle means we lose our potential for movement. Mobilising inside the circle, however, develops an environment to become stable in movement at end ranges. Your brain also has an awareness now of what is possible and can effortlessly define its own midpoint or centre.

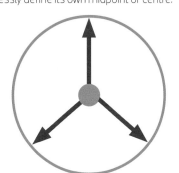

Push the boundaries of awareness with movement

A little old lady with very little comfort zone, for example, can have a life-changing experience when you offer her the chance to explore her own base of support and ask movement of the muscle and joint

How on earth is your body supposed to know where your centre is, when you have no idea what you are supposed to be in the centre of?

WHAT THE FOOT?

In gait the spine is never static either: the foot drives movement at the pelvis, which influences directly motion in the spine

system. I guarantee you that nobody else will have tried this approach, her brain will instantly cotton on to new possibilities and the frail little frame will grow and expand into life again – just following this model.

DOES THE MODEL WORK IN UNDERSTANDING ADAPTATION?
In a perceived centre environment, the dot represents our perception of centre and the limitations that come with it in the system. For example, we could be right-side dominant and to access the left side of the circle below would require more effort than access to the right side, giving us an indication of the adaptations the body must make.

Our movement is then limited to the shape of the circle, which is distorted by way of whole-body alignment changes thanks to an off-centre centre of mass and also to the size of the circle, since the bigger the awareness, the greater the opportunity for the body itself.

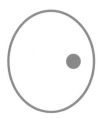 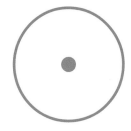

Core stability only arises in its true and natural sense when there exists full mobility in the system and the body gains awareness of the full-range potential in the three-dimensional joint system as a whole.

It's the same for the knee and the ankle. Stabilising the ankle and knee by limiting its movement

potential is not a solution for the brain to perceive optimal movement in the knee or the ankle. It, too, has its own base of support and centre of mass that must explore and 'know' its full range in order to develop the stability it requires.

Would you rather be the dot? Or the circle and the dot?

Should 'core mobility' be the new paradigm for working with injury and strengthening the bridge between the torso, the legs and the arms? I think so. I also find it more fun, less exasperating, more effective and it has an instant impact on all who take it on.

THE SPINE
In this sense, in order to explore the circle, the spine cannot remain neutral. The muscles that attach onto the spine, according to the big rules of movement, are all set up to decelerate spinal motion away from its neutral position – away from the dot inside the circle. To get the muscles to work we must therefore have to take it away from its neutral position, away from stability and into mobility.

In gait the spine is never static either: the foot drives movement at the pelvis, which influences directly motion in the spine.

Through the six phases of the flow motion model, you will notice that the spine should flex and extend twice per stride, go from full left rotation to full right rotation and laterally flex from right to left, going in the opposite direction to the transverse plane, with a scoliotic shift along the way.

WHAT THE FOOT?

WHERE'S NEUTRAL?

Neutral is the point that the spine passes through on its journey from left rotation to right rotation whilst simultaneously passing from left lateral flexion to right lateral flexion. At this moment the spine will be upright. This moment occurs in the transition phase of gait.

There is an interesting phenomenon, however, in that at this moment the spine is flexing through the swing phase and thus is never neutral and extending at the same time.

There is NEVER a moment in walking gait where the spine exclusively extends: extension will always be coupled with a rotation and a lateral flexion, **but will never couple with neutral.**

Even efforts to attain neutral spine in the conventional model – which is already flawed – fails further when we realise that an upright spinal column in everyday movement will be coupled with a flexing spine. Any attempts to extend the spine in neutral should be coupled with rotational and lateral flexion movements, too.

There is a desperate requirement from the people around us to begin to grasp that it is no longer about neutral spine; it is not about core stability and it is not about isolating and localising things down to find out what is wrong.

It's time to teach the body to explore its own possibilities by looking at and assessing exactly what the body does on a day-to-day basis and comparing that to what it is designed to do all the time.

FLOW MOTION, FASCIA AND CORE MOBILISATION

In summary, movement is simply an experience of mass management – or, put another way, how you manage your mass. How you manage your mass is a daily challenge; for many people it's really tough, favouring one leg or taking short strides to get the job done. Balance, stance and dynamic flow motion are all reliant on successful management and mobilisation of your mass.

Your centre of mass lies at L4/L5 in the lumbar vertebral column. Movement of this structure impacts on everything and faulty movement here can have disastrous consequences. In gait, the kinetic chain begins with motion at the calcaneous and is optimised by contact of the big toe, and the communication up the whole chain demands movement in each and every joint. My second big rule – joints ACT and muscles REACT – suggests that gait is symbolised by skeletal movement and controlled or managed by the soft tissue system, also known as muscle or fascia. Movement around our central point, in particular the pelvis, spine and ribcage, signifies that muscle such as our 'core' or deep abdominal muscles are also reacting to skeletal movement. In this sense, all soft tissue is managing human movement in reaction to skeletal motion first.

Fascia is inseparable in its function. To stretch it is pointless: to mobilise it is key. How do we mobilise it? Through effective and optimal movement of the skeleton in relation to the gait phases of the flow motion model. How do we manage the fascial system in a squat or yoga-based down dog? By exploring the base of support around that squat or down dog position, in effect challenging the position of the centre of mass over the base of support.

WHAT THE FOOT?

*In effect,
our bodies
learn to be
stable through
movement*

Same for gait. All movement is a challenge of what is available in the structures required to complete the movement. In many cases it's all of them.

Core stability or core mobility? For me, that's a no-brainer. The body works by experiencing movement and in the event that it cannot be optimal, it downgrades the performance of the body whilst ensuring that daily goals are achieved. Where pain is present, the body naturally inhibits movement somewhere and facilitates movement elsewhere. It's called compensation and what we find is that parts of the body become too stable and others too mobile. The only time it works is when there is an even distribution of both stability and mobility at the same time.

This way of looking at the body highlights the need for BOTH stability and mobility in the system. What's most interesting is that the body and brain actually learn to be stable through a mobile approach. Exploration of the end range, and challenging the base of support, enhances our awareness of the eccentric, isometric and concentric ranges, making us stronger in each. With stability, in actual fact, taking place at the edge of your movement potential, the greater the eccentric load, the stronger the concentric contraction and the more stable the isometric moment must be – ultimately, the more stable we will be throughout the whole dynamic range as well.

In effect, our bodies learn to be stable through movement. Movement is the only method available to the body, recognised by the brain, to increase the ranges, challenge our perception of what is optimal and to develop stability in this fully mobile system. Not stability at a midpoint, but stability over

the whole range of movement without ever having to spend hours needlessly training your TVA. Yes, your body does need to be stable as it moves, and its ability to be so is determined through the quality of the movement. As we slide more to the stability end of the spectrum, we start to lose mobility, and yet as we focus on the mobility end of the spectrum, we begin to enhance stability, too. I find it really interesting. Try it...

Here are some ideas for challenging core mobility: **www.whatthefoot.co.uk/coremobility**

I ran these past a Pilates workshop once with simply a four-point position for before and after reference. My favourite feedback in the moment of experiencing the 'after' position was "I'm afraid to say it, girls... but he's right!" Feel this in action, experience it, challenge your base of support and join the revolution.

CASE STUDY

I worked with AP (not an acronym for Anatomy and Physiology!) to resolve a double disc herniation problem. His therapy had basically been based on the side of the coin that promotes stability – localised care with the goal of minimising his movement to protect the back.

His gait was lumbering, flexed forward, and his movement around the lower back and pelvis was minimal. Stability and minimisation was working – at least the goal of shutting it down was being effective, but AP was experiencing no relief for his pain.

He could not believe the impact of one session on his mobility and his pain, integrating pelvic and foot motion whilst teaching him the desired role of the pelvis and the ribcage. He felt amazing, but wasn't out of the woods. This was an extremely tall man who would have to do his homework – but I knew he would since he had already placed so much value on the movement patterns and had felt the benefit of them. Session two and his limited motion had been completely unlocked by his commitment and the strength of the exercises he had been prescribed. However, I discovered through the course of the session that he could not mobilise his pelvis in the sagittal plane, so I referred him to a chiropractor friend of mine who was able to assist with that part of the process: Dr Carlyle Jenkins of Harley Street. AP said that he could not believe that I was the first person ever to discover this and that I was also the first therapist he had ever seen who freely referred out to another practitioner – this I found quite odd! When AP came back to see me a week later, he had new movement and freedom in his pelvis, which I set about integrating into his whole system – ensuring lines of communication between the foot, spine and shoulder girdles were well and truly open! In the third session we began exercising and moving his body in ways he had not done before. This continued through the fourth session, by which time AP was out of pain, standing tall. Double disc hernia to full mobility in four weeks, and I'm talking lunges, squats, full flexions with rotations and overhead work as well. Did he really have a disc problem? I will never be sure... At the end of the fourth session, however, AP booked in for four more sessions to exercise at the highest level possible and prepare him for the heli skiing trip he had previously cancelled.

Double disc herniation to heli skiing in seven weeks... Now that is not bad going!

We seek political stability, stability in our jobs, stability in our home life, stability in the financial markets and even in our health, and the irony of this is it's 100% impossible. Stability is impossible in a dynamic and mobile world

IN SUMMARY

To summarise the flow motion model, the fascial system in motion and this new idea of core mobility, I'd like to bring huge awareness to the fact that at no point in the process of walking, moving or other 'in motion' activities, is any single part of the human body functioning in isolation.

There is no joint-by-joint approach whereby one joint is mobile and the joint either side is stable. Each joint is moving all the time. Granted, some joints have less motion available to them than others, but there is still motion present, for instance in the lumbar spine, and yet motion in that lumbar spine needs exploring to bring life to the pelvis and the thoracic spine above it – there is a constant flow of communication between all joints as well as all muscles that attach to the joints and the structures around them.

Your core, a structure that, glorified for its stability, is never ever actually stable – not in stance and certainly not in gait. Why stabilise it? Because it ticks the box of the localise, minimise and stabilise model – a model steeped in fear: a fear shared by many practitioners the world over. If it hurts don't move it – yet, ironically, moving it is exactly what the body is crying out for, in fact begging you to do, in an integrated way of course, a way that speaks to the brain, sings in harmony with the nervous system and stimulates the fascial realm to reinstate old and failed movement patterns so as to generate new levels of efficiency and competency in the human system.

No stability, no localised treatment or minimalist approach ever had that response in the body. Deep down, you know that by now. You know that

movement is present in every aspect of life and stability is nowhere. You seek stability in relationships when what you really need is a dance, two people moving together down the path of life, agreeing, disagreeing, good times and bad times. The moment one of you stands still in the vain hope of stability, your partner simply drifts away. Relatively speaking. Even when you are standing still, the world moves around you, ebbing and flowing, to and fro, relative to the movement that surrounds you – you, too, are in a constant state of motion.

We seek political stability, stability in our jobs, stability in our home life, stability in the financial markets and even in our health, and the irony of this is it's 100% impossible. Stability is impossible in a dynamic and mobile world.

Financial markets change second on second relative to millions of transactions taking place the world over. Recessions are natural dips to the highs of life when the markets are in abundance. To attempt to end a recession is an attempt to disrupt the flow of life. To bring stability to a country without controlling the people in it and removing its freedom is another great irony of the modern day. The world does not stand still and neither do you.

Hormones, the very things that manage your wellbeing (an area of life where you seek stability), have no static state. They often work in highly complex inter-relationships with other hormones in the body. Testosterone and oestrogen are two simple opposites. When one is high, the other is low; there is a reciprocal relationship. They fluctuate all the time, never static, but operating hopefully within a minimum range either side of the optimal balance state for that person – centre. Out of balance,

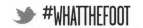

there are disastrous consequences for the human body. High levels of oestrogen, and environmental oestrogens masking as the same hormone, are rapidly becoming known as one of life's biggest killers. This hormonal change is a systemic change that is impossible to pinpoint on the body and treat, so must be addressed globally by treating the system to dig out underlying causes and bring the body back to balance. It must be approached on a higher logical level.

In every 'thing' there is a centre, a point of optimal balance, where performance and opportunity for the 'thing' in question is maximised and optimised. There is also an allowance, a distraction from centre that is deemed as normal. Since centre is a stable point, it is impossible to maintain it, and so the body has an awareness of either side of centre that allows for comfort and wellbeing and the ebb and flow of life. This is the dynamic equilibrium that I mentioned earlier – a place of dynamic balance.

When the human being drifts outside of its normal ranges, things get noticed – physical aches and pains. In society, when the natural balance drifts outside acceptable ranges, things get noticed – sociological aches and pains. The rate of change is the killer: the faster things move away from the dynamic equilibrium, the greater the pain and risk of damage. A huge drop in the financial markets is noticed the world over, and yet tiny drops occur all day every day with no awareness raised at all.

Is it amazing to cross reference the human body with life in this way? I think so. I am consistently fascinated by the 'finding centre' in all things and it has become a wonderful way to view my life, physical and not, on many levels.

I can either act on things to force change or react to change in such a way that I am not left behind by it. I once saw a university student reading a book on Change Management – a book title that made me smile – and the irony is fantastic.

The only constant and guaranteed thing on this planet is change. It happens every second of every day – let me reiterate never stable (just in case you aren't listening) – and the idea of managing change is preposterous. All we can ever do with change is react to it or challenge it. If the book title had said 'Change Reaction', that would have made sense to me.

The irony lies in the teaching of change management, a whole book on it, a whole course on it, a whole career based on it. We are always taught that things will change and in education we are always left behind as things change in front of us. The only way to learn anything, as Sir Richard Branson once said, is "out there in the jungle learning the hard way, learning from your mistakes, learning from your successes, and learning the art of survival: real life versus education – it's the age-old argument".

All I have been discussing and showing you within the five big rules of movement concerns the difference between a contemporary approach to working with the human body (education) versus a new way (real life) that is synonymous with all that Sir Richard has said.

In the model of stability, the knee does not have the chance to make mistakes, nor can it rejoice in its successes and, more importantly, the system around the knee does not benefit from life's biggest driver: survival.

Even when you are standing still, the world moves around you, ebbing and flowing, to and fro, relative to the movement that surrounds you – you, too, are in a constant state of motion

WHAT THE FOOT?

> *The impact on people when you do this will be incredible. Treating a knee until the pain goes away whilst the overall physical compensations remain in place is just another 'accident' waiting to happen*

The educational model has led us down a path of control, stability, isolation and localisation – treating the elbow when it hurts as opposed to digging out the cause and finding a real, long-term solution. The model I am proposing to you – the future, if you like, of your anatomical successes – is based on teaching your physiology the art of survival. Liberating the body, freeing up the systems to work harmoniously through mobilisation, integration and a global (dare I say holistic, meaning 'whole') approach to your interventions.

The impact on people when you do this will be incredible. Treating a knee until the pain goes away whilst the overall physical compensations remain in place is just another 'accident' waiting to happen.

Treating the whole body in an integrated way that eliminates all imbalances and encourages the brain to understand the benefit of working this way overrides all physical compensations as the body re-finds its centre and changes instantly to overcome years of inhibition, liberating the body, effectively making it younger, if younger is determined by what the body can physically do.

As a practitioner reading this book, it's now time to take a look at some of the biggest mistakes made by practitioners when working with their clients who either have pain or don't.

1. Stabilising joints with problems
2. Minimising movement about ANY joint
3. Localising treatment
4. Associating pain with cause
5. Confusing balance with mass management
6. Omitting the feet from any sort of programme or assessment
7. Referring out to therapists who will do any of the above
8. Not utilising movement as a tool
9. Using movement without a full understanding of coupling and integration
10. Not learning the five big rules to the depths that are possible

These mistakes are all based on not seeing and working with the body as a whole system, on a higher logical level. The biggest problem often comes with those practitioners who have bravely stepped into the new world of movement – mainly personal trainers and coaches – but who have not yet developed the full understanding of coupling and integration.

Mobilising the abdominals in an upright position is all well and good for tone and muscular benefit, yet such movements could have phenomenal impact on the brain and nervous system if the complete coupling of the joint system was simultaneously present.

Done correctly, mobilisation of the abdominals (all tissues between your pelvis and ribcage) could be your ticket out of back pain, providing integration in the feet and shoulders along with the abdominals and low back muscles is present, to manage the point in the back that is painful. Failure to couple the body correctly could lead to greater areas of tension and compression that will either a) continue to hold pain present or b) fail to encourage the brain to utilise the new range of awareness and thus find centre.

It is this area of coupling that is KEY and that is being OVERLOOKED in the new wave of movement education. Throwing fascial lines around in a three-

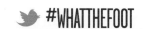

dimensional way may sound like one way of getting the body out of its comfort zone, but there are limitations to that as well if we cannot integrate the fascial line as it was designed to be integrated into movement, according to the five big rules and the six flow motion movement patterns created by a true understanding of what is happening in gait.

Once again, you are probably wondering why I can't give you all the answers here and now in the book. Well, as I have said before, I am results driven and the idea of sending you out into the world to cause chaos and not peace is not on my agenda. As you may know, or will have guessed by now though, is that there is a very deep and detailed way of learning how to work with the human body in motion in this way.

WHAT THE FOOT?

CHAPTER 8: NOW IT'S YOUR TURN

"The only source of knowledge is experience."
Albert Einstein (1879–1955)

I am assuming some level of anatomy here, so don't worry if you struggle with it. Once again, experience of it creates a greater understanding than words on a page.

I think I'd like to leave you with the opportunity to look at some things and hopefully see them differently as a result of reading the book.

Let's call it a reward for sticking with it and getting this far. I'd like to give you a couple of things to take away with you and look at with your clients/patients tomorrow.

MUSCLES
Let's take a look at three different muscles in the body and get beneath the role that each muscle plays in the body.

Let's look at the psoas major, a muscle much scrutinised for its imbalance and impact on the physical and emotional components of the body. We'll look at the abdominal muscles, since everyone has a bizarre and desperate need to know them better, and we'll look at the rhomboids or lower traps, without which spinal extension would not be possible – and since in the majority of people spinal extension would appear impossible, it stands to reason that we might benefit from taking a look at the rhomboids and lower trapezius muscles.

Remember big rule #1? Muscles lengthen to contract. In essence, this means that muscles BOTH lengthen and contract. So we have to, when looking at any muscle, first work out where it starts, where it stops (origins and insertions), before then looking at the following things:

- What anatomical motion is the muscle set up to decelerate?
- In which plane does it act to decelerate that motion?
- In which triplanar position does the muscle have no option but to contract?
- What other muscles are working to decelerate the same joint or set of joints?

PSOAS MAJOR
Origin
Transverse processes of T12–L5 and the lateral aspects of the discs

Insertion
In the lesser trochanter of the femur

Muscle action – sagittal plane
As discussed previously, the psoas is known as a hip flexor, unsurprisingly because its primary action is to flex the hip. That is a sagittal plane motion. Which position, though, does the psoas access most flexion from? This is how we begin to really determine the role of the muscle – in particular, if muscles do lengthen before they contract in motion.

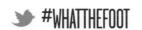

If flexion is the primary action of this muscle then it should make sense that it is set up to decelerate extension in the sagittal plane. Put another way, it flexes during the motion of extension to slow down the extension action. This is the eccentric role of the psoas muscle.

To give the muscle full contraction potential – that is, a full range of flexion – it makes sense to put the hip into full extension prior to the contraction of the muscle. Fully extended means the psoas muscle has no option but to contract to flex the hip back towards the central midpoint of its motion.

A – When I sit somewhere between flexion and extension, I have the option to either flex or extend.
B – When I sit at full extension, I have no option but to flex.

Of course, it's not just about the hip, since the psoas muscle attaches onto the spine as well. This suggests that not only does the muscle flex the hip, but would serve to flex the spine as well. Once again, it pays to consider that it is therefore also set up to slow down spinal extension. If, once again, spinal extension is not present in the body, this impacts upon the psoas since it cannot achieve full lengthening in motion, and this ultimately limits the range available to the hip and subsequent joint interconnections.

If you now have a look at the other planes, I'm interested to see what you would come up with.

Frontal plane
In the frontal plane, notice that the psoas insertions obviously do not change, but it's the actions of the structures that impact upon it (joints ACT, muscles REACT).

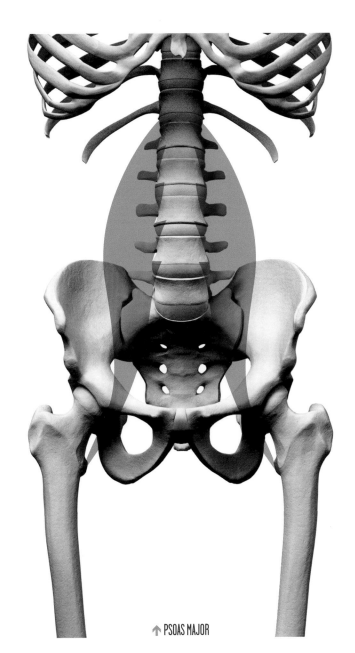

↑ PSOAS MAJOR

WHAT THE FOOT?

So what motion is available to the hip joint in the frontal plane?

_____

And what motion is available to the spine in the frontal plane?

_____

Now consider where the muscles actually attach again and in which direction the hip and spine would go in order to trigger a decelerative reaction in the muscle. Look again at the image of the psoas muscle on page 165 – which way would the spine go to lengthen the muscle in the frontal plane and which way would it go to shorten the muscle in the frontal plane?

	Lengthen	Shorten
Hip		
Spine		

Answers available =
Hip: adduction OR abduction
Spine: left lateral flexion OR right lateral flexion

Transverse plane
Similarly, address the muscle in the same way for the transverse plane.

What motion is available to the hip joint in the transverse plane?

_____

And what motion is available to the spine in the transverse plane?

_____

NB: Remember that there is only one spine, so it cannot rotate internally or externally – it can only rotate one way or the other (left or right). Believe it or not, this is a common mistake!

So which direction would the spine rotate to cause a lengthening of the psoas and initiate a decelerative reaction?

	Lengthen	Shorten
Hip		
Spine		

Answers available =
Hip: internal OR external rotation
Spine: rotation away from OR rotation towards the psoas in question

Now can you put it together?
To put it together, you simply make sure you are standing up and place one hip (one psoas muscle) into the position that you have written down for both the hip joint and the spine in each plane where muscle lengthening is taking place. And, finally, work out how to get the muscle from fully lengthened to fully shortened and back again – you are now moving the psoas in motion.

Clue: to get hip extension you put the opposite foot forward (left foot forward to get right hip extension, stretching the right psoas).

Go online here to get the answers once you have had a go at figuring this out:
www.whatthefoot.co.uk/psoas

🐦 **#WHATTHEFOOT**

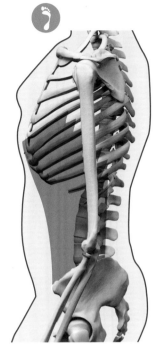
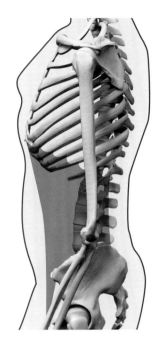

THE ABDOMINALS
(Rectus/internal and external obliques)

Origin

Rectus abdominus: pubis symphysis

Internal oblique: inguinal ligament, iliac crest and lumbodorsal fascia

External oblique: ribs 5–12

Insertion

Rectus abdominus: costal cartilage of ribs 5–7, xiphoid process of sternum

Internal oblique: linea alba, pubis and ribs 8–12

External oblique: iliac crest, pubic tubercle and linea alba

Now, I know that many of you will probably start thinking that the rectus abdominus isn't a transverse plane muscle and, equally, the oblique muscles aren't sagittal plane muscles, and some of you could find it hard to visualise this muscle in any plane other than that of flexion and extension.

Let me ask you though, what do you think happens if there is straight sagittal flexion or extension? Do you think the oblique muscles simply switch off and are not involved? No, of course, there must be some action taking place as two structures move towards each other or further apart, mustn't there? Likewise, in pure rotation, if there is such a thing, there would have to be some adaptation in the fibres of the rectus abdominus for the movement to take place.

Notice in the image on the right that there is very little difference between one muscle and another and there is little doubt that a spinal rotation would

← LEFT TO RIGHT: RECTUS ABDOMINUS, EXTERNAL OBLIQUE, INTERNAL OBLIQUE

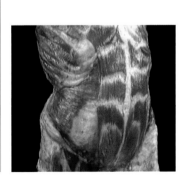

cause fibres to move with the movement, thus there can be a transverse appreciation of the rectus muscle and sagittal appreciation of the oblique set.

Muscle action – sagittal plane

For movement purposes, you can simply consider this abdominal set of muscles to be one. As you are going to be looking at the ribcage and pelvis, we safely assume that any movement of these two structures will generate a lengthening or shortening reaction in the abdominal muscles.

Once again, knowing the attachment sites, we should be able to determine that motion of the ribcage and pelvis directly impacts upon the abdominal muscles.

We all know that a sit-up is a concentric contraction of the abdominals, but what else can the abdominals do and what other value can they bring to our bodies?

Answer the questions again:
- What anatomical motion is the muscle set up to decelerate?
- In which plane does it act to decelerate motion?
- In which triplanar position does the muscle have no option but to contract?
- What other muscles are working to decelerate the same joint or set of joints?

Do this by firstly asking:
What motion is available to the pelvis in the sagittal plane?

_____

And what motion is available to the ribcage in the sagittal plane?

_____

So having worked this out, check the muscle attachment sites again and work out in which direction the pelvis and ribcage would travel in order to trigger a decelerative reaction in the muscle.

	Lengthen	Shorten
Pelvis		
Ribcage		

NB: For the ribcage, consider it operates like the pelvis with an anterior and posterior tilt in the sagittal plane, laterally flexes in the frontal plane and rotates in the transverse plane.

Answers available =
Pelvis: anterior tilt OR posterior tilt
Ribcage: anterior tilt OR posterior tilt

Frontal plane
What motion is available to the pelvis in the frontal plane?

_____

And what motion is available to the ribcage in the frontal plane?

_____

Now consider where the muscles actually attach again and in which direction the pelvis and ribcage would go in order to trigger a decelerative reaction in the muscle.

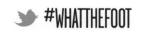

Tip: Think of the abdominal muscles as one unit and focus on one side, i.e. the abdominal set on the left-hand side of the spine (linea alba).

	Lengthen	Shorten
Pelvis		
Ribcage		

Answers available =
Pelvis: opposite hip hike OR same-side hip hike
Ribcage: left lateral flexion OR right lateral flexion

Transverse plane
What motion is available to the pelvis in the transverse plane?

And what motion is available to the ribcage in the transverse plane?

Now consider where the muscles actually attach again and in which direction the pelvis and ribcage would go in order to trigger a decelerative reaction in the muscle.

	Lengthen	Shorten
Pelvis		
Ribcage		

Perhaps worth considering here that shortening in the transverse plane can only be from end range back to centre, as past that point, the lengthening will begin again.

Answers available =
Pelvis: left rotation OR right rotation
Ribcage: left rotation OR right rotation

Now can you put it together?
Find a place where you can get the most lengthening and shortening out of your abs. You'll find that standing up gives a different feel to your abdominal work – flexion virtually does nothing for your abs in this environment. But can you maximise it and where would you maximise it from? Where is the point of most contraction?

Finally, work out how to get the muscle set from fully lengthened to fully shortened and back again – you are now moving the abdominals in motion.

Your movement experience should also portray that, when moving the pelvis and the ribcage in such a way, you'll notice you are having a major impact on the movement of your spine. It's easier to understand this way, and the intricacies of the spine fall into place when the mobility of the pelvis and ribcage are enhanced.

Go online here to get the answers once you have had a go at figuring this out:
www.whatthefoot.co.uk/abs

WHAT THE FOOT?

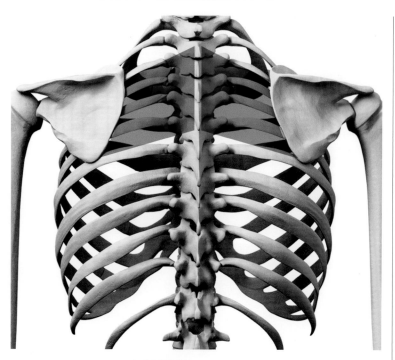

↑ RHOMBOIDS

RHOMBOIDS

Origin
Spinous processes of T2 to T5 vertebrae

Insertion
Medial border of the scapula

Muscle actions — sagittal plane
This time we are looking at the spine and the scapula — two structures that are so closely connected without being connected at all! Any motion of the spine causes movement in the scapula and vice versa.

Flexion of the spine always causes a protraction, abduction and elevation of the scapula, with extension of the spine causing the opposite. If you

are unsure about this, put your hands on someone's scapula and ask them to slump. You will feel them glide upwards and outwards. I often refer to the glide upwards and outwards as a pronation of the scapula and the glide downwards and inwards as a supination of the scapula. Again, supination being the extensor dominant action that optimises our postural influence.

So, same questions again:
- What anatomical motion is the muscle set up to decelerate?
- In which plane does it act to decelerate motion?
- In which triplanar position does the muscle have no option but to contract?
- What other muscles are working to decelerate the same joint or set of joints?

Do this by firstly asking:
What motion is available to the spine in the sagittal plane?

_____

And what motion is available to the scapula in the sagittal plane?

_____

Having worked this out, check the muscle attachment sites again and work out in which direction the spine and scapula would travel in order to trigger a decelerative reaction in the muscle.

	Lengthen	Shorten
Spine		
Scapula		

🐦 #WHATTHEFOOT

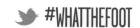

WHAT THE FOOT?

Answers available =
Spine: flexion OR extension
Scapula: elevation OR depression

Frontal plane
What motion is available to the spine in the frontal plane?

_____

And what motion is available to the scapula in the frontal plane?

_____

Now consider where the muscles attach again and in which direction the spine and scapula would go in order to trigger a decelerative reaction in the muscle.

	Lengthen	Shorten
Spine		
Scapula		

Answers available =
Spine: lateral flexion away OR lateral flexion towards rhomboid in question
Scapula: adduction OR abduction

Transverse plane
What motion is available to the spine in the transverse plane?

_____

And what motion is available to the scapula in the transverse plane?

_____

Now consider where the muscles actually attach again and in which direction the spine and scapula would go in order to trigger a decelerative reaction in the muscle.

	Lengthen	Shorten
Spine		
Scapula		

Answers available =
Spine: rotation towards OR rotation away from rhomboid in question
Scapula: protraction OR retraction

Now can you put it together?
So, if you were looking to get the rhomboids to react by lengthening to create an improved extended posture, where would you take them first and what might this look like following the joints ACT and muscles REACT approach?

Finally, work out how to get the muscle set from fully lengthened to fully shortened and back again – you are now moving the rhomboids in motion.

Go online here to get the answers once you have had a go at figuring this out:
www.whatthefoot.co.uk/rhomboids

Once again, it's a simple way of pointing out that isolation of a muscle, if you want to integrate it into movement, is a futile gesture

WHAT THE FOOT?

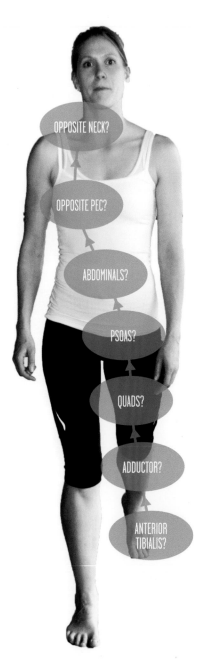

OPPOSITE NECK?

OPPOSITE PEC?

ABDOMINALS?

PSOAS?

QUADS?

ADDUCTOR?

ANTERIOR TIBIALIS?

THE FINAL QUESTION

Worth considering is this final question I have posed:

● What other muscles are working to decelerate the same joint or set of joints?

When the psoas is in its fully lengthened state and thus acting to decelerate the hip as it reaches full extension, it would pay to notice that other muscles, too, are involved in decelerating the movement as a whole. Obvious muscles are those that also generate flexion from extended positions, such as rectus femoris, sartorius and quads, to name a few.

We also looked at the role the hip flexor plays in controlling the motion of the spine, and you should have noticed that it is the same as the abdominal muscles. Is the psoas an abdominal muscle?

Whatever your thoughts on this last question, this does mean though, that the psoas and the abdominals play a role together to manage the extension of the hip and spine, and since we noticed that the thigh muscles must also contribute to deceleration of hip extension, we have crossed a mass expansion of muscle tissue that serves to manage that moment, and it only goes further as you travel down into the foot and up into the shoulders.

Once again, it's a simple way of pointing out that isolation of a muscle, if you want to integrate it into movement, is a futile gesture.

The rhomboids, however, would appear to oppose the action of the abdominals and the hip flexors, as they are set up to decelerate flexion in the spine. Does this mean they inhibit each other reciprocally?

In an optimal functioning body, the psoas and the rhomboids will match each other with perfect timing – as the hip extension and spinal extension change direction, so must the psoas and the rhomboids take on an opposite state of contraction:

In motion:

Hip extension and spinal extension = psoas lengthens and rhomboids shorten

Hip flexion and spinal flexion = psoas shortens and rhomboids lengthen

Whereas in a squat – a fixed movement – the rhomboids and the hip flexors must shorten simultaneously to allow the hip flexion and spinal extension to take place.

In squat:

Hip flexion = psoas shortens and rhomboids shorten

Hip extension = psoas lengthens and rhomboids remain shortened

So there is reason to believe that muscles are set up only to react to the physical skeletal state. They effectively do what they are told relative to the goal of the movement and the intention of the person in that movement. Add to that a compromised system, either posturally or with range limitations, and the action and reaction of muscles changes again.

So?

So if all stands true, and muscles and joints have a relationship that is completely dictated by the intention of movement – where both muscles and joints function optimally when they can access both the optimal centre point whilst experiencing the extremes of movement – then it should also stand true that the only thing to do is to get to grips with this material. The five big rules present a very real case that is not currently fully addressed in most walks of anatomical education. When I look at the current ways of working with the human body I maintain one thing: that pain remains unsolvable when we think in a conventional and traditional way.

My mission is to change that way of thinking, and I hope that just by reading this book you have begun the process already. Allow yourself to think differently. Question what you see and reflect on the material when working with clients.

- Is a tight muscle really short and tight?
- Does it really need stretching?
- Why is it tight in the first place?
- What is happening in the person's body and movement that is making that happen?

For instance, a short, tight psoas is most likely a hip joint that can't attain full range because of a variety of factors in the whole kinetic chain. Most likely there is a relationship down at the foot, which could simply be that the same-side big toe cannot achieve 60° of dorsiflexion. If that is the case there is NO point in stretching or foam rolling the psoas out again and again and again...

...and again.

What's more, if a rhomboid shows symptoms of being tight, but is clearly in a lengthened state, you have two options:

i) to concentrically shorten it by bringing the scapulae together

Pain remains unsolvable when we think in a conventional and traditional way

WHAT THE FOOT?

ii) take the opportunity to initiate big rule #1 and lengthen the muscle further so it has no option but to contract. You would do this by further flexing the spine and protracting the shoulders. Sounds unconventional? Good, because it is...

One of these is to follow the new rules of movement and the other is to adhere to an old paradigm that limits what is possible. I'll leave it for you to decide.

Oh, and next time you think a hamstring needs an old-school stretch, please think again.

It's time to think bigger, ask better questions and combine your existing knowledge with the knowledge available from movement anatomy, and get even more outstanding results with yourself and your clients.

Missing link

The great thing about AiM is that it takes on a life of its own in the hands of different practitioners; an osteopath will use it differently to a physio, who will use it differently to a PT, who will use it differently to a yoga teacher. Yet each one reports back just how powerful a tool it is to have in your practice, clinic, studio or gym. Many have described it to me as the missing link; the process that links together the conventional approach with a real grounded result, normally backed up with the following type of conversation:

"I can't imagine why I never considered the overriding gait patterns as an influence that would keep the pain coming back. As soon as I was in a position to recognise the failing patterns and reintroduce them to the body and the brain, it had the potential to minimise the imbalances and tension-compression

relationships in the whole body. The body would truly find centre."

Tom Morgan, an osteopath, wrote an article for *Osteopathy Today*. I summarise his closing points of the article in the boxout below as the natural benefits to you and your work – in this case though, specifically for an osteopath. The whole article can be found online here:
www.whatthefoot.co.uk/osteotoday

"SPECIFICALLY, THIS IS WHAT IT HAS DONE FOR ME:

● **My understanding of human motion and how each phase of the flow motion model impacts on each joint and soft tissue in the body has transformed the way I work with the patient.**

● **I am able to restore movement patterns that the body is failing to use to improve overall function.**

● **I do many osteopathic techniques 'in motion' that are effortless to do and I find them more effective than static ones.**

● **I offer effective three-dimensional exercises for patients that work. Unlike traditional exercises, these are exercises that get you out of pain quickly. It's a quick win for patients and so they do them at home, too.**

● **I now get people out of pain quicker and for longer using this approach with osteopathy.**

> So when I am now asked what makes me
> an osteopath, I'm confident in saying that I
> examine and treat the body as a whole, from
> head to toe, both on the couch and in motion.
> It's made me a more complete osteopath with
> happier patients."
> (Tom Morgan, Osteopathy Today, November
> edition 2012)

From my point of view, you can replace the word 'osteopath' with your own chosen profession or title, and you will find the same outcome when you incorporate the flow motion model and working in motion into your own practice – whatever that may be. If you consider what you were taught in the educational establishment that awarded your profession as one side of the coin, then the value you can add to that qualification by pursuing the other, more elusive motion–based side of the coin, is, as reported by many, priceless.

Ultimately, much of what I have said has been to discuss the body, the anatomy, the physiology, etc. What I want to discuss – something we pursue at a much higher level through the educational process – is the role of the nervous system and the overriding power of the brain. There is probably another book in there somewhere and is something that interests me greatly. Working with the body is one thing – working with the brain to influence the body is another. Working in the subconscious realm as opposed to the conscious realm is yet another deeper level for you to look forward to, and since motion underlies our very existence on this planet, you begin to tap into the brain at these depths the moment you start pursuing motion as a clinical tool. What's more, pain is registered in the brain, not in the body parts where you actually feel the pain. As the brain is hardwired to determine the posture that causes your pain in the first place, it might be a useful idea to think about how we challenge the brain's perception of its own body, as opposed to focusing our attention on the parts that make the whole.

This becomes easily accessible when you welcome the five big rules into your clinic or gym, begin to think wholly about the human body, be bold enough to get your clients off the couch or the floor and get them moving. Watch the flow motion model come to life, make pain a thing of the past and reintroduce the world back to its own version of peak performance.

CHAPTER 9: WHAT ARE YOU WAITING FOR?

"Yesterday I was clever, so I wanted to change the world. Today I am wise, so I am changing myself."
Rumi (1207-1273)

The only way to get to grips with new material is to get out there and do it. Play with it, watch it, question it, challenge it and ask it to create winning solutions for you and your clients. Any process like this, i.e. a whole new way of looking at the body, should start with you, working on yourself; and when you are sure there are obvious wins that you can offer your client, only then should you go ahead and try it on them. My only caveat is that you DO NOT go out and try this on people who are in pain until you have full knowledge of what you are doing. In the right hands the information I have laid before you is an incredibly powerful tool. In the wrong hands it's as bad as any other misunderstood advice out there in the fitness and therapy industries.

You might be thinking that it's not safe to flip the anatomical model upside down and expect to get results. I get that. Let me suggest something to you, though. When you walk, you follow the five big rules of movement. When you run and jump, you do the same. A footballer, tennis player and golfer also operates in motion. What I am not doing is flipping the anatomical model upside down – I am simply relooking at the model and highlighting the parts that have been overlooked and forgotten about for the past 50+ years! It is purely an extension to all the knowledge in the industry and research labs and, hopefully, skillfully woven into a fantastic solution for people.

Why don't we see if we can actually see it in action?

Here is a list of 'to dos' for you to go and do today:

Go and watch some people walk
Check for hip and spinal extension and foot resupination. Notice that virtually nobody does any of these things and, as a result, their glutes don't work and their hamstrings are long and tight.

Assess your client's feet
Go on, take their shoes off! Are they flat-footed, high arched, do they look weird? Are they turned out or have bunions? Refer back to page 118 to work out why. Enquire as to whether they ever have any problems in their feet. How do they move when they walk? Can they resupinate the foot? Are they used to wearing orthotics? What patterns can you see running up the body from the feet?

Mobilise the mass and challenge the base of support
In an upright position, the base of support surrounds you. This can easily be challenged by visualising yourself on a clock face.

Stand single-legged in the centre of the clock face and reach the non-standing leg to each point on the clock, challenging the base of support by reaching as far as you can, until you feel unstable. This is the body leaving the comfort zone and where muscles have no option but to react and bring you back to centre. You have just created interconnected awareness in

WHAT THE FOOT?

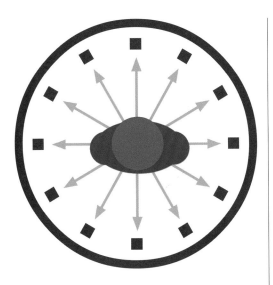

the feet and each and every mobilised joint above. Nothing broke, did it?

Challenge and mobilise the core

This is a chance to play with the spinal gyroscope on page 82 . You can make use of the clock face again in, say, a press-up or four-point kneeling position (**www.whatthefoot.co.uk/coremobility**) or try this in a lunge and single-leg balance position to further mobilise the mass.

Challenge the feet to wake up

Your feet have been dormant for years. What do you have to do to wake them up? How can you give the supporting muscles no option but to contract – the contraction being one that causes resupination of the foot? What position do you have to place the feet in to ensure this happens? Put another way, where do the muscles of the foot supinate from? How many positions can you put your foot in and does anything strange happen when you do?

Do the opposite of what you think you should (in a safe way, of course)

I can guarantee you have a client today whose butt muscles have been asleep for years. Use the big rules to wake it up. Forget extending, abducting and externally rotating it – go ahead and flex it on a step, internally rotate it and adduct it. Try it on yourself first, feel the burn and then gently apply it to your client (again remaining in a pain-free environment).

In this sense, there is a final piece of advice if the rules are going to play a huge part going forwards in your life:

If it extends, flex it, and if it flexes, extend it! This goes the same for the other planes of movement, too.

And the final caveat once again is:
DO NOT WORK WITH PEOPLE IN PAIN UNTIL YOU LEARN HOW TO DO THIS FIRST-HAND AND ARE TAUGHT BY ME OR ANOTHER AiM GRADUATE TEACHER.

If it extends, flex it, and if it flexes, extend it!

CHAPTER 10:
WHAT'S HOLDING YOU BACK?

"Patience you must have my young padawan."
Master Yoda

It's different
I've seen it before: a bunch of macho trainers who adore their mirror muscles, struggling to get into the whole-body movements. They probably felt silly and, yes, full-body movement can sometimes look more like a dance than an exercise, until, that is, you can do it whilst throwing a 20kg weight around your head. Which is absolutely possible with regular access to it... naturally.

If you aren't used to whole-body exercise and unconventional movements, use them with a view to getting yourself out of your comfort zone and recognise that, actually, nobody is watching you, has ever watched or even gives a shit about what you look like in the way you thought they did. Get over it.

This is a tool that will change not only your body and your client's body forever, but will change your business as well in a huge and dramatic way.

Stability seems to have worked up until now
If you have seen success with the stabilisation model then it's highly likely that you have been controlling your client's pain as opposed to expressing the freedom in the body of the client. You have created an internal environment that has adapted to the pain by stabilising as opposed to creating a new way of

functioning in the body that, in effect, reverses years of compensations and adaptations.

Stability works when there is a need to generate a comfort zone in a client's body. Once there is an element of comfort zone in place, even where pain is present, the barriers created by the comfort zone need smashing down so the body itself can experience growth and advancement by challenging its own limitations and inhibitions.

Once you step outside of your own comfort zone and recognise that there is enormous value in the world of stability AND mobility together, can you then fully embrace the human form? Remember that stability is a key component in the human body. I haven't once said it's bad, I have merely suggested it is bad where mobility is not present. Stability is the isometric part of the curve that occurs in between the concentric and eccentric actions. Stability lives on the outer edge of our metaphorical base of support whilst mobility resides inside it and is the driver of the whole system. Mobility generates stability and thus the two can never, and should never, be separated.

It won't work for me
If you are thinking that this way of looking at the human body won't work for you and your clients then I can only encourage you to experience it yourself before jumping to that conclusion.

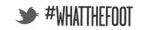

WHAT THE FOOT?

Both myself and many AiM students have had success with everyone from young children up into the 90 years+ category, from double herniated discs to athletes whose careers are on the line due to not performing.

There are AiM graduates who began the programme three months out of completion of their Personal Training qualification who have been able to offer help with back, neck and knee problems right there on the gym floor without the need to move on to a referred practitioner (which is always recommended in cases where more help is required, of course).

Imagine that the client never has to leave your care to get back to full training and, in many cases, you'll find them limping on the treadmill having seen everyone and stuck for a solution. They simply crack on through the pain in a desperate bid to get fit and lose weight whilst slowly getting worse.

In less than half an hour, the client can feel the difference, and have a glimmer of hope that maybe they don't actually need to spend their life in pain and that, YES, maybe there is actually another solution.

It works for everybody and that includes you.

It's too complex
The traditional way of looking at anatomy on the one side of the coin is often deemed simple in its isolation and minimalist way. Far easier is it to look at the knee and break down the components of the joint, whilst getting to grips with each and every muscle and the action it imparts on that joint, than to address the impact of every joint in the body on the knee and the muscular chains that wrap around the body, managing each and every movement.

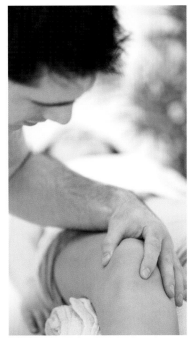

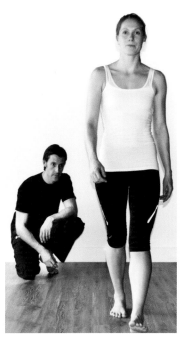

Yes, it seems highly complex at first, but so was driving when you first learned to do that. When you stop looking at the body with a laser and pull back to look at it under the light bulb, you will see the body so much more clearly. You'll see it in a way that makes clear sense as to why the knee might hurt in the first place.

Examining the knee is complex; looking at the body as a whole is simple. It takes me the duration of the course to convince students of this, and they all get there in the end — some earlier than others, but that's OK.

The complexity comes in the detail of the joint. A plethora of pathologies arise with the many failings

Examining the knee is complex; looking at the body as a whole is simple

WHAT THE FOOT?

The speed of results that you will get with yourself and your clients creates a need to know more and understand better the practice of movement as a therapy

in its movement patterns. Simplicity comes when we learn the value of teaching the whole body to find centre; to reorganise itself in such a way that all the pathologies drop away.

An example of this is medial knee pain. An assessment shows alignment problems, and muscle testing shows inhibited and facilitated muscles with weak, tight and dominant tendencies, and joint testing highlights inhibited range.

Under the light bulb, drawing back from our attention on the knee, you notice an over-pronated foot that collapses too quickly in motion on the same side as the knee and a pelvis that is rotated away from the affected knee.

Under the laser you choose to treat the knee, massaging muscles, strengthening and stretching them, mobilising the joint in the open chain and with strong consideration to move in and operate.

Under the light bulb you choose to enhance the function of the foot, challenge the awareness and stability of the foot, ankle and knee with movement, whilst simultaneously addressing the range and movement in the hip, too. Once the hip and foot are in perfect optimised communication with each other, you have your solution, as the knee must fall into line, in series with the foot, ankle and hip.

Under the laser, the massage and stretching continues without the intervention of movement as the client walks away from each session over-pronating, limping and replaying the old pattern that caused the medial knee problem in the first place.

The simplicity arrives at challenging all of the joints to get out of their comfort zones, communicate with each other and together find a new centre of potential.

The AiM course has been designed to give you full access to understanding the body and simplifying the process of working with the human body — eliminating the complexity for you and for the client.

Watching your pennies?
There are a host of courses and workshops available to the hoardes of personal trainers and therapists to upgrade skills and improve techniques as well as develop new ideas. Most all of them are set in the traditional way of thinking, on the conventional side of the coin, and are simply repackaging what you already know.

Most of them are amazing, but, sadly, some of them are not.

In my experience so far of working with trainers and therapists, they all come away from the first part of the AiM programme with a spring in their step (physically and metaphorically) and guaranteed new tools, as well as a brand new way of looking at the human body. This goes for everyone from the personal trainer to the chiropractor.

The amazing thing about this method is that it acts as an extension to everything you know, or can be used as a stand-alone method. Either way it adds simplicity and power to each and every session you do.

The speed of results that you will get with yourself and your clients creates a need to know more and

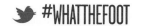

understand better the practice of movement as a therapy. Rapidly, word of mouth will spread and there will be a queue of unsolvable problems at your door. In order not to be overwhelmed by work and become the ultimate irony – a knackered and unhealthy therapist – you will have to put your price up to ease the demand.

To bring human movement into your clinic or practice is to virtually guarantee results, and attract great referrals and excellent relationships with co-practitioners who you can send work to and from. It has to be this way so that your work can put the icing on the cake of other therapists, and you, too, when you are struggling, or unsure, can refer out as well. Your care and attention given to your clients will be second to none and your understanding of their predicaments will be paramount.

Real tools, real professional relationships and, more importantly, real results fast, is the key to growing your business and standing out in a sea awash with therapists and trainers who are all doing the same work.

It's time to stand out from the crowd in your area.

I don't believe you
If you have got this far in the book and still don't believe the message I am conveying, I urge you now to read back to the case studies and absorb the reality of each situation, and how, prior to connection with me, each case had been deemed unsolvable by a host of practitioners.

Knowledge of one side of the coin, the conventional side, renders such cases unsolvable. Knowledge

of both sides of the coin made each case solvable and the results were quick, effective immediately and long-lasting.

www.whatthefoot.co.uk/testimonials

"So what, exactly, has Gary done?"
This question is often raised when students discuss their work and my work with a conventional therapist.

The experience for the student is that Gary solves people's unsolvable pain and teaches others to do the same by looking at the anatomy and figuring out exactly what it does in motion; the patterns it creates throughout the kinetic chain and matching them up with the patterns that should be created through the kinetic chain.

When we break old patterns and replace them with new ones, the pain disappears and the client moves into a new dimension where training again for anything is now possible.

The reaction of the therapist is either a) "Wow, that sounds interesting. How can I learn more?" or b) "So what, exactly, has Gary done?"

Question b) is designed to challenge my credibility and so I thought I'd tackle it upfront right here in print.

No, I do not have a degree or qualification in physiotherapy, osteopathy or chiropractic. I did a three-month course to become a personal trainer and a sports therapist. Prior to that I worked on and serviced ski boots in the Alps, in France, learning and studying the anatomy of the foot.

WHAT THE FOOT?

**I pride myself
on describing
exactly what
the body does
and not what
we think it does**

When I began training people years later, it was obvious that nobody was talking about the foot as an important factor in training movement, and certainly there was little awareness that a lack of mobility in the foot could lead to pain in the shoulder.

So I began to integrate the two and finally learnt to watch the body and connect the dots up the whole body.

In answer to the question "So what, exactly, has Gary done?", I simply say that I have spent years watching and studying the human body and the movement patterns it creates. I have looked at joints and the biomechanics of each joint. I have looked at muscles, their attachment sites, and laughed at the muscle actions cited in the anatomy book. I have worked with chiropractors, osteopaths and many trainers and specialist coaches to make sure my knowledge is razor sharp and I have always applied this to the moving body. When Tom Myers released a book on fascia I was overjoyed to see how the fascial model and the flow motion model overlapped, bringing huge clarity and sense to the world of fascia in my brain and to the world of movement in others'.

I pride myself on describing exactly what the body does and not what we think it does. For example, we think the rectus abdominus flexes the spine, but in an upright position it does not – not in the traditional way anyway. Gravity flexes the spine when we are upright. What I notice is that the rectus abdominus controls the amount of extension available in the spine and flexes when it needs to, to bring it back to centre. In order to get an abdominal workout I suggest you extend your spine, in this case, as opposed to flexing it. The difference in abdominal tone and abdominal (including core) functionality is amazing.

So it is that this idea of describing purely what the body does took over my life in such a way that the old ways of training people died off. Sure, we all like a bench press and a good squat, but even that pales into insignificance when you fully understand the three dimensionality of the pecs and the role it plays in posture and the body. It's just a matter of trialling new ways of movement to truly challenge the pecs in a bench press, for example – and, personally, I find it more fun, a deeper muscular sensation and greater connectivity throughout the torso so I can feel upper back muscles, pectoral muscles, lats and abdominals all involved in a bench press workout... It's just a matter of joining the dots.

Looking at the joint system in this way proves also insanely valuable. None of the students I have taught have an awareness of what one motion in the foot can have on the hip, for example. Yet when you understand the biomechanics (complexity stripped bare), it becomes so clear that what the industry thinks is happening at the hip and what actually is happening at the hip are different.

The result of this way of investigating the human body means that we start to tap into the neurological circuitry and patterning of the brain. What's truly fascinating is that the brain knows exactly what it wants from the human body, knows exactly how to optimise itself and what is the most efficient opportunity for that body. We, as practitioners, have absolutely no idea – we only think we do.

So when I started working with Oliver Dudley in 7in7on7, I had no idea what his body needed or what processes I was going to go through. All I could do was literally ask the body to feed me the information that I needed to know so that I could point him in the

WHAT THE FOOT?

right direction. I have the tools, but it's his body that will make the final choice as to whether to be healthy or not come the time to run, run and run some more.

Movement is all about giving choice to the brain, creating a new habitual way of movement, stance and being that is far superior to the alternative.

When you ask what Gary has done, the only accurate answer is that he has created a system to observe, study and optimise human movement by spending hours in the pursuit of understanding what exactly it does. The system is taught in such a way that you yourself are gifted the opportunity to work it all out yourself, guided by the practitioner, so as to cement the process in your own brain. The hardest part of the process will simply be forgetting some of the hard and fast rules you currently believe to be right!

TO END ON THE RIGHT FOOT

"There is no secret to this life — our grasp of it just lies beyond what we know in a world few are willing to explore." **Gary Ward**

How should I conclude this book? A summary, an overview, or perhaps better to bring the two sides of the coin back together? As I said right at the start of this book, I once heard someone say there are three sides to every story: "his version, her version and the truth!" The same goes for a coin: heads, tails and the edge it stands on — or balances on.

The two sides of the coin are brought together by this third edge, making it real, giving it substance. A head without tails has no integrity. Likewise, in science, a single-minded viewpoint has no integrity without a counterargument. This is why I know that if more people were to entertain the dual side of the coin, we could begin collectively to move towards the truth of how the human body works. There are still too many factions preaching their knowledge, steeped in evidence founded purely on the basis of a science that is drenched in one-sidedness.

My way of addressing this was to look at what the body does, when it does it, how it does it and, finally, why it does it. By sharing with people what is really happening, I managed to override the brain patterns of what those people think is happening. It's even a lot of fun (for me) and incredibly taxing for them. I've had physios say "all those years at university, wasted!" I've had people declare they want to reject the information as it conflicts with everything else that they have paid good money for!

My first response is NOTHING is wasted. Your journey to this point so far has been perfect — dare I say, 100% functional? The great thing now for that physio is he can easily bring the two sides of the coin together and I hope this means he can work at a higher level with the body, too, working in integrity and in truth.

I began the book with my rants and raves. The common point with each rant is that each is based on the one side of the coin. Stretching comes to mind instantly. Of course, stretching is a component of movement, it's just not meant to be held statically or in a single dimension. Sure, osteopathy takes place on a couch and disregards the joint interconnection through the chain in motion, but imagine the power of being able to do that, get somebody off the couch and integrate the adjustments through movement. Weight training in a single plane? Hogwash? Not really. If it's a movement, a human movement nonetheless, then there is a good chance it will influence the body and brain positively. If the squat is a new movement pattern, for instance, it would benefit the brain and the nervous system in so many positive ways.

My point is that, having parked what you know at the beginning of the book so as not to obstruct your thinking during the book, now is the chance to bring it back in and fuse the two together. AiM is not a technique per se. It's a concept, a philosophy that is not devised to overrule existing methodology, but to add to it. To make something more of it or to help you understand on a deeper level that which you already know.

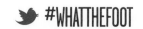

WHAT THE FOOT?

Sure, it evolves the way you work, but so did the iPad. Evolution is part of life and it's a natural progression in life to build on all that has gone before. We've run out of stuff to research on the conventional side of the coin. Ironically, the only way to go with research is inwards, more local, more isolated, and we have effectively been running ourselves into a corner.

"The problem with research – the more we know about less and less until we know everything about nothing!" I heard Paul Chek say this. I'm not sure if it's his original quote or not, but it made complete sense to me. Evolution is built on change, challenging the very base of our knowledge and what we know. Growth and development of anything springs out of the same environment. Challenging the current paradigm in such a way can only have one outcome: change, adaptation, liberation. A perceptual shift towards centre or, as I like to describe it, towards the truth.

Mobility and stability. Isolation and integration. Challenge and support. Eccentric and concentric worlds. A fusion of all this will ultimately show itself as the truth in how this body of ours works. It most likely won't look like I expect it to look either, as with all evolution it will eventually take on a life of its own.

Like the people we work with, how can we know what is optimal for them when the thing that ultimately determines what is optimal, the brain, actually resides in the person seeking to make the change? We can't. We apply our philosophies, facilitate movement as it was designed, and ask the body to adapt in such a way that it heals the person or moves them towards their true version of centre. We as practitioners can merely provide an environment for that healing or development to take place.

A big problem not just in our industry, but in the medical industry as well, is that people are coming to you with a 'fix me' attitude. They place their care in your hands. If you think about that for a second, that is one hell of a responsibility to take on, in particular when they are the ones who choose to change or not...

This philosophy is all about tackling the idea of creating an improved environment for movement, which requires a whole-body adaptation to alignment, a whole nervous adaptation through plasticity and whole awareness shifts as to what is possible in a body that leads us to a pain-free and high-performance outcome.

You are not the healer, you are not the reason your clients and patients get results. You are merely a facilitator, a messenger on the road to success. You are and can only be a healer of your Self.

You are a facilitator. The methods you apply are received by your clients/patients and the outcome is determined by their brain and their own nervous system. To get bigger results requires more choice, more movement and more newness – newness that restores your old forgotten patterns, the loss of which have led to today's inhibitions.

I regularly ask students what their definition of centre would be. My favourite response, by Sean O'Leary, KMI and AiM practitioner, is:

"Centre is the place where the body has got used to being, which it has adopted through habits, patterns and previous experience, and is intelligently worked out given the internal resources available."

"There is no secret to this life – our grasp of it just lies beyond what we know in a world few are willing to explore."

The finding centre theories run consistent in the physical body as well as the mental, emotional, nutritional and hormonal aspects of the body, too. I'd love to get to grips with those areas, using this philosophy, and get closer to the truth of that, too.

Is it complex? I don't think so. Is it easy to apply? Yes, providing you don't convince yourself of how hard it is, when it isn't! Eighty per cent of the results I have talked about in this book come from exploring new movement, outside of their normal patterns and ranges, whilst keeping within a pain-free environment. For now, why don't you simply go out and try that, without worrying about the intricacies of rapid correction and integration of movement into the whole. When you are ready to move on with that, give us a call at AiM or visit the website and look for workshops and courses in your area. If there isn't anything available, get in touch and we'll make it possible – wherever you are.

Thank you. I am honoured you have taken the time to read my book. I hope you've had some light bulb moments, some 'What the foot?' moments and, more importantly, I hope the book has opened your mind to a simple, powerful and incredibly effective (not to mention rapid!) tool that can transform the way you work with your existing skill set and current client base.

Yours in movement and health,

Gary Ward, 2013
#whatthefoot

THE BEGINNING...

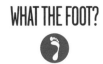
WHAT NEXT?

Whatever your intentions were in reading this book – I hope you have enjoyed and taken something from it.
If you are wondering "what next?" or "what more is there?" ..... I would like to offer you a free download of my next e-book –
"A brief look at pain, neurology and your brain" all you have to do is click on the link....

TO DOWNLOAD IT:

Please visit: www.whatthefoot.co.uk/painbook

For all other Anatomy in Motion information and social media please find us at:

Web: www.anatomyinmotion.co.uk

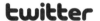

Twitter: @GaryWard_AiM

www.facebook.com/garyalanward
www.facebook.com/anatomyinmotion